Praise for *Spiritual Yoga*

"*Spiritual Yoga* brings Yoga back to its classical roots as a beautiful art and transformative science of Self-realization. Gyandev McCord shows brilliantly how to integrate Hatha Yoga into the greater practice of Raja Yoga and deep meditation. The book highlights the enduring importance of the teachings of Paramhansa Yogananda as one of the most authentic guides for Yoga in the West and for the entire world."

> —DR. DAVID FRAWLEY (Pandit Vamadeva Shastri), author of *Yoga and Ayurveda*, Director of American Institute of Vedic Studies (www.vedanet.com)

"A wealth of knowledge for teachers and students. Highly recommended."

> —LARRY PAYNE, Ph.D., E-RYT500, YTRX, Co-author, *Yoga for Dummies, Yoga Rx & The Business of Teaching Yoga*

"The explosion of interest in postural yoga has improved the health and well-being of millions. Unfortunately, it also threatens to make 'yoga' synonymous with physical fitness, obscuring its deeper and more profound treasures. Gyandev McCord's book is a welcome antidote. By focusing on yoga as a universal repertoire of methods for spiritual realization, it adds a vital element to the growing literature on this ancient science."

> —PHILIP GOLDBERG, author of *American Veda: From Emerson and the Beatles to Yoga and Meditation, How Indian Spirituality Changed the West*

"I served with Gyandev McCord as a co-founder of Yoga Alliance. His integrity and dedication in communicating the deeper essence of yoga in a commercial world is exemplary. He is a master teacher who conveys a profound understanding of yoga through each and every page of this powerful book. I highly recommend this book to yoga practitioners of all levels, as well as to all spiritual seekers."

> —HARI KAUR KHALSA, Director, Hari NYC, author of *A Woman's Book of Yoga: Embracing Our Natural Life Cycles* and *A Woman's Book of Meditation: The Power of a Peaceful Mind*

"*Spiritual Yoga* gives voice to a new era in the understanding and practice of Yoga. Lucid and accessible, it provides an experiential pathway to the ultimate awakening that Yoga offers to everyone."

—Swami Ramananda, Executive Director, Integral Yoga Institute of San Francisco

"*Spiritual Yoga* is a jewel among yoga books. It will take the yogi, whatever his style, to a deeper experience of his own practice. Precious principles for uplifting consciousness are presented with a delightful mixture of authority and lightness. The asanas themselves teach perfect alignment, while leading the yogi to their deeper, inner meaning. I have studied under Gyandev, receiving great benefit, and am certain that the reader of this book will share my experience. I recommend it with all my heart."

—Jayadev Joerschke, Director, Ananda Yoga® Academy of Europe

"Whatever your style of Yoga or spiritual tradition, Spiritual Yoga will deepen your practice—and enhance your entire life. It offers great value for every practitioner, from beginner to advanced. I particularly appreciate the emphasis on the oft-overlooked connection between physical alignment, subtle energy, and higher consciousness. Gyandev McCord has provided a complete guide sure to instruct, inspire, and transport many a spiritual seeker."

—Nicole DeAvilla, E-RYT 500, RPYT, RCYT, author of *The 2 Minute Yoga Solution*, Member of Accreditation Committee of the International Association of Yoga Therapists

"I am extremely happy to see this book. Gyandev McCord covers a wide range of important yogic teachings with clarity and simplicity, rendering it very easy to understand without sacrificing spiritual depth. These are authentic and ancient Indian teachings that will give valuable aid to people all around the world."

—Guruji Dileepkumar Thankappan, President, International Gurukula Community

"In today's crowded Yoga marketplace, the deeper purpose of Yoga is too often lost among the many purely physical approaches. Spiritual Yoga takes Hatha Yoga back to its roots as a vehicle to know a reality beyond the senses. It also offers a comprehensive—and rarely found—treatment of the major pranayama and meditation techniques in simple, straightforward language. Nayaswami Gyandev brings insights from his own deep practice, along with the experience of decades of teaching, into a book that is both informative and inspiring."

> —MURALI VENKATRAO, Director of Yoga Teacher Training, Ananda Institute of Living Yoga

"*Spiritual Yoga* shows how Hatha Yoga is much more than physical movement; it is, above all, a spiritual science. With insight and clarity, Gyandev unifies Yoga's many techniques into a single, consistent approach that anyone can practice. One thing that sets this book apart is its guidance in cultivating—and applying to Hatha practice—the most powerful consciousness-raising tool of all: right attitude."

> —LYNN BUSHNELL, YogaWorks OC Regional Manager

"*Spiritual Yoga* is a precious jewel—I know, because the techniques in this book changed my life. I was broken, heading down a dark path of self-destruction, but through regular practice my heart began to heal. I gained the strength to let go of negative patterns and embrace the possibilities of new and amazing opportunities. Gyandev and his wife Diksha have been more than just teachers and mentors; they are truly the living example all yogis should aspire to."

> —KARI BURGOS, Owner/Director, Inner Harmony Yoga, San Pedro, CA

Spiritual YOGA

AWAKENING TO HIGHER AWARENESS

Nayaswami Gyandev McCord

Crystal Clarity Publishers

Nevada City, CA 95959

Copyright © 2013 Hansa Trust

All rights reserved. Published 2013

Printed in China

ISBN 13: 978-1-56589-272-9

eISBN 13: 978-1-56589-518-8

Cover design by Tejindra Scott Tully

Book design by Molly Heron

Library of Congress Cataloging-in-Publication Data

McCord, Rich.
Spiritual yoga : higher awareness through ananda yoga /
author: Nayaswami Gyandev McCord.
pages cm

"Also on cover: From the Teachings of Paramhansa Yogananda,
author of Autobiography of a Yogi (with his Autobiography photo)."

Includes index.
ISBN 978-1-56589-272-9 (quality pbk. : alk. paper)
ISBN 978-1-56589-518-8 (epub)
1. Hatha yoga. 2. Spiritual life. 3. Mind and body.
I. Yogananda, Paramahansa, 1893-1952. II. Title.

RA781.7.M398 2013
613.7'046--dc23

2013013344

I DEDICATE THIS BOOK—and offer my deepest gratitude—to Swami Kriyananda, and to his (and my) Guru, Paramhansa Yogananda. All that I know of Yoga has come through their teaching, inspiration, and guidance in my own practice.

Table of Contents

5

SIX Meditation   172

6.1—The Science: Concentrate and Calm Your Mind   173

6.2—The Art: Attune Your Mind to What You Seek   178

SEVEN Yoga as a Way of Life   181

7.1—Find Balance   182

7.2—Create a Supportive Environment   183

7.3—Find Freedom in Service   185

7.4—Outer Fitness Feeds Inner Fitness   186

7.5—Dietary Choices Can Help   187

7.6—Lighten Up   188

EIGHT Two More Aids for the Journey   190

8.1—Right Attitude   190

8.2—A Guide for the Journey   192

Foreword
by Swami Kriyananda

More than sixty years ago, my Guru, Paramhansa Yogananda, asked a small group of us to perform yoga postures for a visiting dignitary. Up to then, I was merely an average performer of the yoga postures, or *asanas* as they are called. That day, in my Guru's presence, I found that I could perform all of them perfectly—so much so that from then on he always called on me to perform them, especially when he had guests. After performing them, I served him and the guests lunch. After they left, he and I would sit at the table and converse. Always, he had sage words to share with me, many of which have found their way into my books of his sayings.

From him—not verbally, but by a sort of osmosis—I learned what I know of the postures.

Many years later I lived in San Francisco, working to earn the money needed to create the first of the communities that he called "World-Brotherhood Colonies." I was teaching yoga meditation classes, and soon began teaching classes also in *Hatha Yoga*. I wasn't satisfied with the way the asanas were being taught in America—a sort of "this will slim your hips, girls!" approach that left out of reckoning their real spiritual purpose. Therefore I developed a new approach, which later came to be called, "Ananda Yoga®."

Hatha Yoga is based on the teachings of Patanjali's "eight-limbed" explanation of yoga: not a system, but rather an outline of the universal attitudes and states of consciousness through which every spiritual seeker must pass, regardless of his religion, if he would find God.

Patanjali himself did not actually mention the yoga postures. His third *anga*, or limb, was Asana, which to him meant sitting perfectly still, relaxed, and with a straight spine. Hatha Yoga developed out of this third anga. In my own classes, I emphasized the spiritual benefits of each pose. I showed how various positions of the body can influence right attitudes in the mind. To aid in this process, I wrote an affirmation for each pose that would affect the mind in a direction the pose suggested.

My Guru said to me one day, "Your work in this life will be lecturing, editing, and writing."

"Sir," I replied, "haven't you yourself written all the books that are needed?"

"Don't say that!" he said, sounding slightly shocked.

It was because of those words that I have written all my books. But always I have written them to be seminal. For many years Nayaswami Gyandev has continued the development of this system of Ananda Yoga. I am very grateful to him for popularizing it in America. This book will be a valuable adjunct to the teachings of Paramhansa Yogananda. I wish it great success.

Gurgaon, India
October 2012

Preface

Spiritual Yoga? Isn't that redundant?

Well, yes and no. Yes, because Yoga is—and always has been—first and foremost a spiritual discipline. And it's much more than physical postures; it's a comprehensive system for allying self-effort with divine grace in order to experience the eternal oneness of soul and Spirit.

And no, because not everyone comes to Yoga for spiritual reasons. Many people come instead for physical therapy, or stress reduction, or most commonly, a fitness regime. Increasingly, those needs are being met by specialized approaches that, although they offer many benefits, often omit the spiritual dimension of Yoga.

Now, with spiritual hunger growing worldwide, more and more people are asking, "How can Yoga help meet my spiritual needs?" They suspect that spiritual experience can be cultivated through Yoga practices—and they're right. That's why I've written this book: to show others how to quicken their spiritual growth by skillfully integrating the postures, breathing exercises, and meditation.

In fact, *any* approach to Yoga can uplift your state of mind to some degree. It will uplift you even more if you practice with right attitude, the most powerful spiritual tool of all. And still more is possible if you also cooperate actively with the inner workings of subtle energy and consciousness. Such is the approach in this book. (Right attitude, which we'll explore, is not about moral judgments; it's about what raises consciousness.)

In more than thirty years of teaching, I've seen that *anyone* can practice this way and receive marvelous benefits on all levels: physical, mental, and spiritual. There's no need to be young, or thin, or flexible. Each person can find an expression of this practice that suits his or her condition, abilities, and goals.[1]

---

[1] Certain health conditions call for working with a qualified teacher and/or healthcare professional to modify the practice appropriately.

Although parts of this book are specific to the system that I teach—Ananda Yoga®—all the principles are universal: they come from the ancient Yoga tradition. And happily, many other teachers are exploring these same principles and sharing them with their students. I hope that this book will in some way encourage and support each of them.

Through your ever-deepening practice, may you come to know your own divine essence.

Acknowledgments

I offer my deepest thanks to the generous souls who helped manifest this book: to Barbara Bingham for her many patient hours of photography; to Melody Hansen, Badri Matlock, and Barbara Bingham for serving as asana models (I'm the fourth model); to Kripamayi Caughlan, Monisha Vasa, Maitri Jones, and many others who offered valuable feedback on earlier versions of the manuscript; and to Prakash Van Cleave and Richard "Dayanand" Salva, whose many insightful suggestions markedly improved the clarity of presentation.

Introduction

Imagine that you've hired Michelangelo. You've heard that he's a good painter, and you want him to repaint your kitchen cabinets. Plain white. No doubt he would do a great job, but might you be missing out on something much better?

It's the same with Hatha Yoga, the physical branch of the greater science of Raja Yoga. If you practice only for its physical and psychological benefits—increased flexibility, strength, and vitality, reduced pain or stress, and so on—you'll receive some of those benefits, but you're likely to miss out on something much better! For Hatha Yoga is above all a tool for spiritual growth. Its highest purpose is to help you raise your consciousness and achieve ever greater, ever more unshakeable happiness.

Can mere bodily positions and breathing exercises do that for you? A little bit, yes, but much more is possible if you know how to amplify the effects of these practices through the hidden powers of your mind and heart. This book shows you how. If you're new to Hatha Yoga, you'll find here instructions to begin a safe, enjoyable practice that will raise your consciousness. If you're experienced, you'll find many ways to deepen your practice by working more directly with energy and consciousness—and I hope that you'll be patient with any explanations intended for those who are newer.

Our springboard will be Ananda Yoga®, one of the many spiritual expressions of Hatha Yoga. Ananda Yoga comes from the teachings of Paramhansa Yogananda, author of the spiritual classic, *Autobiography of a Yogi*. He was the first great master of Yoga to make his home in the West, where he dedicated his life to sharing India's ancient spiritual wisdom and techniques. His direct disciple, Swami Kriyananda, developed the Ananda Yoga system, based on Yogananda's approach to spiritual practices (see Appendix A: Origins of Ananda Yoga).

Ananda means "bliss, divine joy." Union with divine joy is thus both the literal meaning and the highest aim of Ananda Yoga. Although it also brings many physical benefits, our focus here will be on the psychological and, even more, the spiritual benefits.

In Ananda Yoga, you work directly with the body's *prana* (energy, life-force) to heighten your awareness as well as to achieve greater relaxation, vitality, and overall wellness. The practice includes three kinds of techniques:

- *Asanas* (postures/poses)
- *Pranayamas* (energy-control techniques)—These include breath-control techniques, *bandhas* and *mudras* (physical actions that help direct the flow of energy in the body), and Paramhansa Yogananda's Energization Exercises (see Appendix B: Further Exploration). For clarity in this book, "pranayamas" will refer only to breath-control techniques.
- Techniques of meditation, the central practice of all Yoga

We'll explore all three areas, as well as ways to blend them together into a revitalizing and uplifting practice.

The Only Source of Knowledge

Spiritual Yoga is a quest to know a greater reality—beyond the senses, intellect, and emotions. Your concept of that reality might be cosmic: Spirit, Higher Power, Truth, God, Divine Mother. Or it might be very personal: soul, Higher Self, your own highest potential. Or it might be something else altogether. Yet for every spiritual seeker, the goal is the same: to *experience* that greater reality. Belief can't take us there. Although belief can motivate us and guide our efforts, it is not knowledge—and if we cling dogmatically to belief, it can *keep* us from knowing. Experience is the only source of knowledge.

Paramhansa Yogananda put it simply: "The yogi must turn his *conceptions* into *perceptions*." Another great yogi, Swami Vivekananda, said, "It is no doubt a blessing to be born into a religion, but it is a misfortune to die in one." Both were urging people to go beyond belief and religion into direct, personal experience.

In this book I'll use a variety of names for that greater reality, in hopes that personal beliefs—yours or mine—won't get in the way of knowing. Whatever names I use, dear friend, please substitute your own preferred name. Let's move together into ever-deeper personal *experience*.

The Bigger Picture

Although this book is primarily about techniques, Yoga is much more than that. It's a complete system of living that can be practiced by anyone, anywhere. Techniques alone cannot bring the highest spiritual attainment: Self-realization, the blissful, enduring experience of your inherent oneness with all that is. They can, however, lift your consciousness and give powerful support to all your spiritual efforts, as you'll discover through your own practice.

Terminology

Throughout this book, the first occurrence of each Sanskrit word is italicized, followed by its English meaning. The Sanskrit names of individual asanas, pranayamas, bandhas, and mudras are capitalized; for easier reading, they're never italicized. For an audio pronunciation guide to the Sanskrit words, visit AnandaYoga.org.

See the glossary in the back of this book for explanations of common Sanskrit words, specialized yogic terminology (e.g., ego, superconsciousness, subtle gravity), and some terms pertaining to physical anatomy and kinesiology.

Chapter
ONE

The Art and Science of Hatha Yoga

Yoga is an art as well as a science. It is a science, because it offers practical methods for controlling body and mind, thereby making deep meditation possible. And it is an art, for unless it is practiced intuitively and sensitively it will yield only superficial results.

— PARAMHANSA YOGANANDA

Hatha Yoga, like its parent discipline of Raja Yoga, is a science. Why? First, it's based on universal aspects of human nature. Second, it focuses on direct experience, not on beliefs. Third, anyone who performs the Hatha experiment will receive predictable benefits.

Ah, but how much benefit will *you* receive, and how quickly? Here's where the art of Hatha Yoga comes in. As in any field of endeavor, the outward aspects of Hatha practice will, by themselves, bring only limited benefit. Many people know the techniques of artistic painting, for example, yet only those with deep inner understanding of how to apply those techniques can paint on the level of a Michelangelo. In business, the most successful people have an intuitive *feel* for their products or services, and for the needs of the marketplace. It's the same in art, sports, science, literature, farming, music—you name it.

Similarly, to receive the most from Hatha Yoga techniques, you need certain inner tools and understanding to work effectively on subtle levels of your being. The practices in this book will help you develop those inner resources. To begin the journey, let's get more specific about the science of spiritual Hatha Yoga.

1.1—THE SCIENCE:
MIND-ENERGY-BODY CONNECTION

Every day, you experience part of the scientific basis for Hatha Yoga: your state of mind causes certain movements of energy within your body, and those movements in turn affect your bodily position. It's simply body language.

For example, disappointment, lethargy, and gloom cause energy to flow downward in the body, away from the brain. That flow in turn influences your posture: you'll tend to slump, as if closing yourself off from life. The very words you use reflect that downward movement: "I feel down," or "I feel low," or "I feel depressed."

On the other hand, happiness, enthusiasm, and inspiration cause energy to flow upward toward the brain, which then comes alive. You straighten up into an expansive, life-affirming posture. You tend to inhale as if to embrace the world—and you smile. Your words, too, reflect that upward flow: "I feel on top of the world," or "I'm in high spirits," or "I'm feeling upbeat."

You've certainly experienced all this, even if you haven't seen it as a chain of influence: mind affects energy, which in turn affects the body.

The Key Insight

The reverse is also true: through bodily position you can lift energy toward your brain, and that will in turn uplift your state of mind. This simple insight is a cornerstone of Hatha Yoga, and you can easily prove it to yourself:

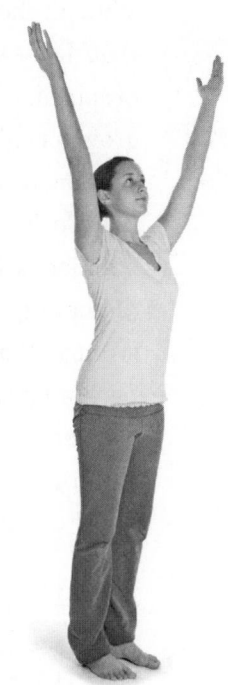

Exercise: On a scale of 1 to 10, rate your current state of mind: 1 is lousy and 10 is terrific. Now set this book aside and stand up.

Stand very erect, with your chest open. Reach your arms overhead, bringing your body into the shape of the letter "Y." Gaze upward. Reach your entire body upward in the direction of your gaze. Inhale smoothly and deeply, hold your breath, and smile broadly. Stay in this position for a few moments, then exhale with a hearty laugh and relax your arms back down into a normal upright standing position. Breathe naturally.

Now rate your current state of mind once again. I'll bet that you've moved higher up the scale—and if you put a lot of energy into it, maybe off the scale.

Think about it: all you did was make physical movements. This is not rocket science. Quite the contrary: it's so much a part of us that we usually pay scant attention to it. That's why we don't realize its power. Imagine what can happen when you *do* pay attention to it, and when you add the power of your mind and energy—as you will in later chapters. Fasten your seatbelt!

By the way, you could (although who would want to?) adopt a bodily position that would move you down the scale. All you need to do is slump, exhale strongly, gaze downward, and frown. And if you keep on doing that . . . well, please don't.

These are very simple examples of the effect of the body on energy and consciousness. Yoga offers many techniques that use the body to lift energy more powerfully than this— and the more energy you lift, the more you'll raise your consciousness. As you'll see in later chapters, each of Hatha Yoga's many asanas and pranayamas has its own special effect on energy and consciousness. You can weave these techniques into an overall practice that brings abundant, calm, focused energy to the brain. That will uplift your consciousness, preparing you for Yoga's most powerful tool: meditation.

The Heart Plays a Role, Too

With all the emphasis on bringing energy to the brain, you may wonder, "Does this mean that the heart isn't important, spiritually[2]?" No, the heart is vital, for it guides the process of spiritual growth from beginning to end. The heart is the source of all desire, and spiritual growth begins with the desire for true happiness. The heart is also the seat of intuitive perception, through which you will experience the ultimate fulfillment: realization of the Self.

Unfortunately, the heart also presents the biggest spiritual obstacles, for it's the seat of emotion, attachment, and desires for self-gratification. These tendencies agitate the heart, disrupting our intuitive perception. They can pull energy downward or outward more strongly than the techniques can lift it inward and upward. They can distort the mind's perceptions, skew decisions, and keep one small and self-centered.

Overcoming these tendencies is the very essence of spiritual growth. In his classic text, the Yoga Sutras, the ancient sage Patanjali writes, "Yoga is the neutralization of the whirlpools of likes and dislikes [which are centered in the heart]." Another great scripture,

---

[2] In this book, "heart" always refers to a chakra (energy center) located near the physical heart. For now, think of "brain" as another energy center, located in the physical brain. As Chapter 2 explains, however, the physical brain corresponds to more than one chakra.

the Katha Upanishad, promises, "When all the desires of the heart fall away, the mortal becomes immortal, and attains Spirit."

How to overcome those tendencies? Certainly not by suppressing them. That would be unhealthy—also futile, says the Bhagavad Gita, Yoga's foremost scripture. Rather, yogis seek to improve their emotional reactions and release attachments, so as not to reinforce those tendencies. At the same time, they seek to increase, calm, and redirect the energy of the entire body—especially the heart—toward the brain. This helps lift the heart out of the turmoil of emotion and desire, and raise consciousness. It also creates in the brain an energy magnet that will help lift even more energy.

Overcoming those tendencies is a big job, and techniques alone aren't enough. They *can*, however, greatly aid your efforts if you take your practice beyond its mechanical aspects—into the art of it.

1.2—THE ART: GOING BEYOND TECHNIQUE

Although the mind and heart can cause trouble, they also hold keys to a deeper practice, and to a deeper spiritual life generally. For among their many faculties are six that are especially helpful for overcoming the downward or outward pulls on your energy and consciousness. Let's explore those faculties and practice a simple illustrative exercise for each one.

Willpower

Willpower is the ability to direct energy to achieve a desired goal. Paramhansa Yogananda called it "the dynamo of all our powers." True willpower is much more than brute force or grim determination. Those attitudes lead to tension, which limits the amount of energy you can muster. Much more is possible. Yogananda declared that in one ounce of your flesh there's enough energy to light the city of Chicago for a week. (Okay, he said that in the 1940s, but that's still a lot of juice!) And the energy of the surrounding cosmos is virtually unlimited.

How to access more energy? View willpower as enthusiastic *willingness*, which is more powerful than forcefulness because it releases energy blockages, opens you to receive more energy, magnetically attracts energy into your body, and helps you cooperate with a greater reality. It's a lot more fun, too.

Many years ago when I was new to Yoga, I participated in a workday at Ananda Village, the ashram where I now live. It was a very hot day, made hotter by the fact that my job was to carry old, rotten lumber—often crawling with carpenter ants—from a dismantled house, up a steep hillside to a blazing burn pile. I worked determinedly, but by mid-afternoon, I was fading.

Then I noticed a woman who had the same job as I, yet she still had a spring in her step. I thought, "Hold on! I'm bigger, stronger, and younger than she is—and I'm in better shape, too. Why am I tired and she's not?"

I observed her for a time, and I could feel that she was practicing willingness, not mere determination. I could also feel that she really had to focus to keep that attitude, but she was doing it. She had *decided* to enjoy the not-so-pleasant work, and that enjoyment was flooding her with energy.

I gave it a try—and I discovered that it wasn't hard. It was also a lot more fun. Now for *your* exercise.

Exercise: Stand up and come onto the balls of your feet, with your arms horizontal in front of you, palms facing up. Bend your knees into a semi-squatting position, as though sitting on the edge of a stool. Keep your torso either vertical or tilted slightly forward from the hips. Breathe naturally and hold this position. When your legs begin to tire, practice your willingness: decide to enjoy being in this position, be enthusiastic about it, look forward to holding it even longer—and watch the energy flood into your body to help you. Fun, huh? Well, it's fun as long as you're willing; after that, it's hard work.

Concentration

Success in anything requires a steady, focused flow of attention and energy toward the task at hand, not giving in to distractions. That's concentration. Most people view concentration as an act of self-discipline, squeezing one's attention very narrowly onto some task. That's a lower form of concentration, because tension is involved, and tension itself will eventually distract you. It's not much fun, either. There are better ways to stimulate concentration.

One way is to bring energy to the seat of concentration: the forefront of the brain, just interior to the point between the eyebrows. That increased energy will stimulate the faculty of concentration and make it stronger. You can also develop concentration by cultivating interest in, or curiosity about, the object of your concentration:

Exercise: Sit upright, close your eyes, and begin to watch your breath. That is, feel it and concentrate on it—without controlling it—as it flows in and out through your nose. Don't analyze or mentally describe it. Simply watch it. For most people, this isn't a particularly fascinating thing to do. After a few minutes—or perhaps just a few breaths—your mind might say: "This is boring. I can breathe without paying attention to it. After all, I do it all day, every day. I'll think about something else instead." End of concentration.

To stay focused, **decide** to be interested in the breath, even fascinated. Observe it with relaxed yet compelling interest. Be intrigued by the breath without analyzing it. You might have to exert a bit of energy to fuel your interest, and that's fine. When you have a high level of interest, concentration becomes natural—and much more enjoyable. **Decide** to be interested.

Feeling

True feeling is not emotion; it's a direct experience of the essence of something. It's an intuitive knowing that's beyond intellect, beyond sensory input—and beyond all doubt. You simply know. We've all had that feeling many times, and if you can clearly remember such a time, you'll recall that the feeling of certainty was centered in your heart, which is the seat of intuitive perception.

Such feelings don't happen only by chance; intuitive perception can be developed. In fact, it *should* be developed, for it's through intuitive perception that you'll someday know your own soul-essence. You can begin by calmly *attuning* your heart to whatever you wish to perceive more deeply. It might be a friend's needs, or a solution to a problem, or how to perform some task. Or, as in the following exercise, energy:

Exercise: In this book, I'll frequently speak of the value of perceiving and controlling energy. If energy seems esoteric, it's only because it's so familiar that we don't notice it, just as we usually don't notice the air we breathe. With a small shift of attention, it's easy to feel energy.

Sit or stand upright, arms relaxed at your sides. Inhale deeply, hold your breath and tense your entire body—squeeze hard—then exhale and relax. Do this several times, until you feel calmly energetic. Now you're on the wavelength of energy, so it's easier to perceive energy. (Couch potatoes aren't on that wavelength, so the only energy they're likely to perceive is the negative energy of resisting activity.)

Close your eyes and turn your attention inward, to the interior of your left arm. With an inhalation, slowly lift your left arm to horizontal in front of you, and stretch forward through your fingertips. As you do so, try to perceive—with your heart—the life-force streaming out through the arm to cause the movement. As you slowly exhale and lower the arm, try to feel life-force relaxing back through the arm, away from the fingertips. Repeat this several times. Yes, you'll also feel such physical sensations as muscles tensing, but try to feel a subtler level beneath the physical. That's energy. (Chapter 2 offers more exercises to help you perceive energy.)

Visualization

Accomplished yogis consider visualization to be a valuable spiritual tool, and they practice in order to develop it. Picturing something in your mind's eye is only part of visualization; even more important is to imagine clearly, strongly, and confidently how it will *feel* in your heart. In other words, create inwardly the total experience you wish to have. The more vivid and engrossing the inwardly created experience, the more it will support your outward efforts. Visualization is a super-tool—a blend of willpower, concentration, and feeling.

You can use visualization to help control energy, a skill that's invaluable in many asanas and pranayamas in Ananda Yoga®. The next exercise has two parts: you'll use visualization to help you feel energy, then to control it.

First, some background: As I touched on earlier, when you inhale, energy flows up through the torso—specifically, from the tailbone up to the medulla oblongata (at the base of your brain), then forward and up to the prefrontal lobes of the brain, just interior to the point in the forehead between the eyebrows. As you exhale, energy travels back down that same route. In fact, Yoga teaches that these movements of energy *cause* inhalation and exhalation. Let's work with that:

Exercise: Sit upright with your spine straight, close your eyes, and breathe smoothly and deeply.

Part 1 (feeling energy): Your torso tends to straighten up as you inhale, and relax as you exhale. Notice, however, something subtler in the center of your torso: an upward sensation as you inhale, and a downward sensation as you exhale. That's energy. If you don't yet feel those sensations clearly, use the torso's slight physical movements as aids to imagining those sensations. Visualize the currents moving along their path from tailbone to medulla to prefrontal lobes as you inhale, then back down again as you exhale. This harmonizes your attention with the energy currents, making it easier to feel the currents. In addition, you've brought your attention into the center of the torso, and energy flows where attention goes. With more energy flowing, you're more likely to feel it.

Even if you **can** feel the energy flowing, it's good to visualize it, because that makes the experience stronger and clearer.

Part 2 (controlling energy): Inhale deeply, then exhale fully so energy returns to the area of the tailbone. Before the body needs to inhale again, strongly visualize energy rising from the tailbone area. Don't try to inhale; just visualize energy rising. If your visualization is strong enough, energy will indeed rise, causing your body to inhale before it needs to. You're controlling energy.

Another example: Inhale deeply, then exhale fully so energy returns to the area of the tailbone. Let the body inhale when it needs to, but at the same time, strongly visualize energy flowing downward toward the tailbone. If your visualization is strong enough, energy will indeed go downward, stopping your physical inhalation. Again, you're controlling energy. Easy! (This exercise is merely to show that you can control energy. Don't make a habit of blocking your inhalations.)

Positive Attitude

These days everyone knows the psychological value of positive attitude; it also has spiritual value as another super-tool for lifting energy and consciousness, and for countering downward pulls. To practice it, don't just *think about* a positive attitude: *have* that attitude, and *express* it in everything you do. That's a good way to strengthen the attitude within you. Here's another way:

Exercise: In Ananda Yoga, each asana is accompanied by an affirmation that reinforces and amplifies a specific positive attitude that the bodily posture can promote. Repeat the affirmation multiple times as you hold the asana, going deeper and deeper into that positive attitude. This is not only an enjoyable experience; it also gives you valuable support for having—and holding onto—that attitude.

With this in mind, let's revisit the exercise for willingness: stand up, come onto the balls of your feet with arms extended in front of you, and enter the semi-squatting position. This is the first phase of Utkatasana (Chair Pose), the affirmation for which is, *"My body is no burden, it is light as air."* Repeat the affirmation mentally, over and over, with enthusiastic conviction.

Through the affirmation, try to connect with the light-as-air **energy reality** of your body, rather than feeling the body only as flesh and bones. Absorb yourself in that freedom from bondage to gravity—not only the body's freedom from physical gravity, but also your mind's freedom from all heaviness, lethargy, and inertia.

Devotion

Devotion is not sentiment or wishful thinking; it's your hunger for truth, your heartfelt commitment to your highest aspirations, the vital fuel for your inner growth. Devotion is your spiritual want-power, and like all desire, it's centered in the heart. Devotion will sweeten your spiritual life and help your energy and awareness rise naturally. Try to infuse it into each of the other five faculties: willpower, concentration, feeling, visualization, and positive attitude. Then your efforts will be strengthened by the unlimited power of the heart.

How to do that? Make devotion more than just a reason for practicing; let it guide *how* you practice. When you put want-power into your practice, every technique becomes more powerful and brings you closer to realizing your aspiration. And if the mechanics of a technique distract you from that focus, keep coming back to it.

Exercise: Sit upright and close your eyes. Feel your heart's desire to realize your highest spiritual aspiration. Strongly offer that desire upward, so that your heart surges upward. Keep feeling that upward surge as you begin to watch the breath, just as you did in the visualization exercise.

Be deeply interested in the breath—not mere curiosity, but a compelling interest born of knowing that you can experience the Divine if you're still enough and listen sensitively enough. Make watching the breath a loving invitation to your Higher Power. Such devotion-driven interest deepens your concentration and infuses any technique—asana, pranayama, meditation—with the unlimited power of your heart.

The bottom line: although methodical, scientific efforts alone can raise our awareness somewhat, we can do much more if we bring these six faculties skillfully into the practice. Then Hatha Yoga comes into its own as a tool for spiritual growth.

Different faculties will be more relevant at different times. Learning to apply them is part of the art of spiritual Hatha Yoga. This process is creative, fun, and rewarding—and anyone can do it. Although no one can *show* you how to apply these faculties, I hope that the above exercises will give you some ideas. Chapters 4, 5, and 6 offer many more tips to help you develop your own inner understanding of this art.

In most people, these faculties need some training in order to be effective, and as you'll see, Ananda Yoga is an ideal training ground. When you apply these faculties in your practice, you'll not only deepen your practice, but also develop a unique, personal understanding of how to apply them effectively throughout your life. And the more you apply them, the stronger they'll become.

1.3—THE HIGHEST ART

Everything so far—both science and art—has been about self-effort. That's essential, and it can accomplish much: relaxation, clarity of mind, vitality, healing, wellness, and a good bit of consciousness-raising. But if you want the highest from Yoga, there's another important factor to consider. I'll tell you a true story:

Some years ago, a certain master teacher was with a group of his students, one of whom was accomplished in the asanas—and rather proud of it.

Sensing this, the teacher asked him, "Can you do the Half Lotus Pose?"

"Yes, sir," the student replied, and he immediately went into the asana.

"Very good," said the teacher. "Can you do the Full Lotus Pose?"

Trying to appear humble, but in fact being rather proud of his ability, the student performed the asana.

"Excellent," smiled the teacher. "Next, grasp your hair firmly with one hand."

Expectantly, the student did so.

"Now," said the teacher, "pull yourself up off the floor."

The student immediately got the point, and was humbled.

The teacher's point was that while self-effort can accomplish much, it cannot by itself bring Self-realization. You can't lift yourself by your own bootstraps—or hair. As so many great spiritual traditions affirm, divine grace is needed. Swami Kriyananda puts it this way:

> Yogis of both the Hatha and Raja Yoga schools often make the mistake of thinking that spiritual enlightenment depends only upon the efforts of the aspiring devotee—as if by techniques alone one could harness the Infinite! A right understanding of the yoga techniques, however, in no way contradicts the need for *kripa* (divine grace), as the *sine qua non* of the spiritual path.

The good news is, divine grace is always at hand. If it seems absent, that's only because the mind and heart are agitated and distracted. In seeking outward fulfillment, we overlook the greater fulfillment that can come from within. Yoga techniques can calm that agitation and, when guided by our sincere aspirations, help redirect heart and mind inward and upward. The calmer, more positive, and more uplifted we become, the more we're on the wavelength of Spirit, so that divine grace can flow more abundantly into our lives. Grace can come in many forms: It can come as an unseen boost to our own efforts, or as the removal of an obstacle. It also can come as a release from an attitude that has held us back. Or it can come as a resolution of a difficult situation, or at least a much-needed change of perception about the situation.

So practice with Spirit. Try to feel Him or Her (or It, or your Higher Self) with you throughout your practice. If you don't feel that presence, imagine how it *would* feel. Ask God to show you how to practice, then try to feel any guidance that comes. In fact, try to feel God with you throughout your entire life. Create a divine partnership—in your own way, through your own unique relationship with, and understanding of, the Divine Friend. This is the highest and most rewarding art of all. There's no limit to what you and the Infinite, working together, can do.

A right balance between science and art, and between self-effort and grace, along with a living relationship with Spirit—these are central to a spiritual approach to Hatha Yoga. There's no secret formula for the right balance; it's highly individual. You'll find it through your own experimentation—and as you do, a new world of joy-filled possibilities will open to you.

Meanwhile, prime the pump for that outpouring of joy: as you practice, be sure to have fun!

Chapter
TWO

Keys to Practicing Spiritual Yoga

To practice the yoga postures with spiritual feeling is to find that they help to develop that feeling. The yoga postures may thus be seen to be an important aid to spiritual unfoldment. If you enter a pose, not jerkily, but with an inner sense of harmony and peace, the very act of assuming that position can help to develop this bhav, *or spiritual attitude. How you get into the postures, the mental thought that you hold during the practice of them, how you rest between the poses—all of these are important parts of the practice of Hatha Yoga.*

— SWAMI KRIYANANDA

You can tailor your Hatha Yoga in many ways: for improved physical function and comfort, for health and healing, for vitality, for inner peace, for emotional stability. Let's explore how to design a practice that can help raise your awareness.

The core principle underlying such a practice is to withdraw energy and awareness from the periphery of the body into the center (the astral spine), then direct it upward to the brain and focus it at the spiritual eye. In short, *inward and upward.* I'll begin with a few basic aspects of the astral (energy) body.

Basics of the Astral Body

The astral spine is the main pathway through which *prana* flows to the brain. It runs through the center of the body, just in front of the physical spinal column, from the tip of the tailbone to the medulla oblongata at the base of the brain; then it bends forward and up to the spiritual eye.

Within the astral spine are the seven chakras, the energy centers that govern all bodily functions; they both influence and reflect your state of mind. With the exception of the seventh (highest) chakra, each chakra has two magnetic "poles," as physical magnets do.

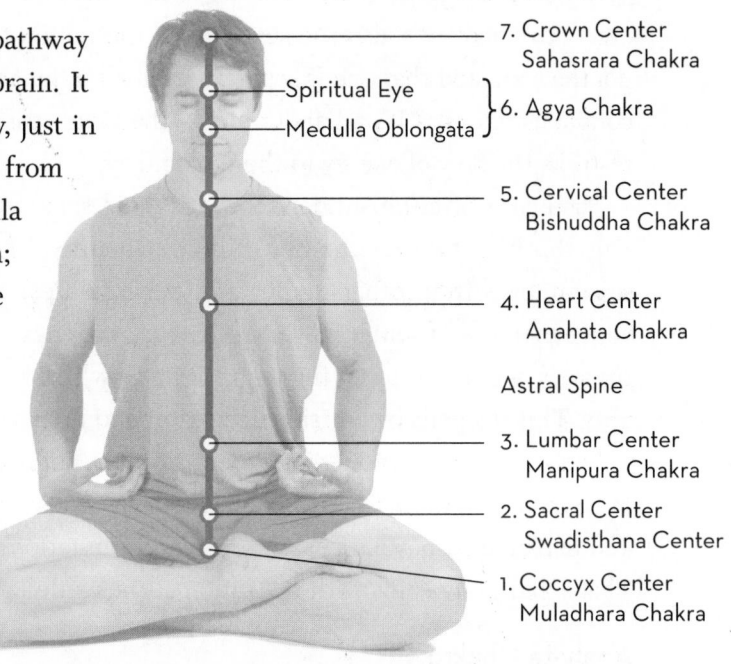

7. Crown Center
   Sahasrara Chakra

Spiritual Eye
Medulla Oblongata } 6. Agya Chakra

5. Cervical Center
   Bishuddha Chakra

4. Heart Center
   Anahata Chakra

Astral Spine

3. Lumbar Center
   Manipura Chakra

2. Sacral Center
   Swadisthana Center

1. Coccyx Center
   Muladhara Chakra

The astral spine with its seven chakras

Agya Chakra

The two poles of the sixth chakra (*agya* chakra) are so distinct that they seem almost to be separate chakras. The positive pole is the spiritual eye, located just interior to the point between the eyebrows in the forehead; it's the seat of willpower, concentration, joy, and superconsciousness. Strive always to bring your energy and awareness to the spiritual eye, not merely to the brain generally. That will vitalize those faculties, lift the heart's energy as well as your state of mind, and speed your spiritual growth.

If you've studied the chakras, you know that all our energy must get to the highest (crown) chakra before we can achieve the state of Yoga (union with Spirit). Then why emphasize bringing energy to the spiritual eye? The reason is that the subtle pathway from spiritual eye to crown chakra won't open fully until we've brought all our energy to the spiritual eye. So that's our first step—and it's quite a big enough step for now.

The negative pole of the agya chakra is at the physical medulla oblongata, where the spinal cord meets the brain. The astral medulla is the primary point through which prana enters the body. It's also the seat of ego: the notion that one *is* the body and personality, not the soul, and that one is separate from all other beings and from Spirit. The more ego-conscious one is—"It's all about me!"—the more tension there is near the medulla, which restricts the flow of energy to the spiritual eye.

The ego is often misunderstood. It's not a separate entity; it's simply the soul mistakenly thinking that it's the body and personality. That identification leads to a sense of separateness from other bodies and personalities, from nature, and from Spirit. Yet a vague memory of soul-bliss lingers in our awareness, calling us to seek happiness. Unfortunately, we seek it by trying to gratify that which we think we are: the body and personality. This deepens our misidentification and takes us farther from soul-bliss.

The yogi seeks to end that misidentification, but not by denying the existence of the ego, or trying to kill it. Instead, he or she seeks to expand that sense of identity beyond the body and personality, beyond separateness and limitation, to the freedom of the Infinite Self. That expansion begins with relaxation at the medulla oblongata.

Anahata Chakra

The other main chakra for the purposes of this book is the heart: the *anahata* chakra. Located in the center of the chest, opposite the physical heart, it's the seat of love, compassion, generosity, kindness, devotion, and intuitive feeling: the faculty with which you'll someday directly perceive your bliss nature. As I mentioned in Chapter 1, calming the heart's energies and lifting them toward the brain, rather than letting them flow downward or outward into emotion and desire, is a central element of Yoga.

Now for some general principles of practice that further the goal of "inward and upward," starting with a few very basic ones that apply to Hatha practice generally (primarily to asanas), followed by others that emphasize a spiritual approach in particular.

Getting Started

- Wear clothing that won't restrict your movement: loose-fitting or stretchy.
- Practice asanas on an empty stomach, at least 2–3 hours after a meal. Some fruit or fruit juice 30 minutes before practice is fine.

- Practice in a well-ventilated area. If you're indoors, it's best to have a window open because fresh air supplies more prana.
- Don't practice in direct sun, or immediately after having been out in the hot sun for an hour or more, or immediately after strenuous exercise.
- Practice barefoot, on a yoga mat if the floor isn't carpeted.
- Don't practice so long that you become tired or dull-minded. You should feel relaxed, revitalized, uplifted, and very awake afterward. You'll gradually become able to practice for longer periods and feel these benefits even more deeply.
- At least occasionally, work with a qualified teacher to get feedback on your technique, and to tailor your approach to your own goals, abilities, and physical condition.

Practice Safely

Hatha Yoga is very safe when practiced responsibly, with common sense. The following guidelines promote both safety and a deeper experience:

- Before asana practice, prepare your muscles and joints to stretch safely by doing simple warm-up exercises that work your muscles and move your joints through their normal range of motion.
- Never impose the techniques on your body; rather, view them and your body as partners in your quest for higher awareness. Practice proper bodily alignment, as explained in Chapter 4. Move slowly and gracefully, with full awareness of what you're doing, and of how your body and mind are responding to what you're doing. In other words, listen to your body and mind—as both a safety measure and an important step toward higher awareness.
- Avoid strain, extremes, and pain. The true goal of Hatha Yoga is to raise your consciousness; it's not a competition, performance, or grueling workout—and injury is the only prize for pushing your body beyond its limits. The minor discomfort of healthy exertion or of a healthy stretch of muscles is beneficial, but if your body signals that you're going too far, or even if you're not sure, back off.
- This book is intended for people whose bodies are basically healthy. If yours is injured, unwell, or vulnerable in some way (including pregnancy), work with a qualified teacher and/or healthcare professional to determine which practices are appropriate for you and how you may need to modify them.

In short, take responsibility for your own welfare. If you don't do that, any physical activity—dancing, housework, sports, gardening—can lead to injury. Consult your health-care advisor before beginning any exercise program. The instructions in this book are not intended as substitutes for medical counsel, nor do they address all physical conditions.

Personalize Your Practice

Modify asanas as needed so that you can relax, maintain safe alignment, and get the most out of your practice. To these ends, Chapter 4 offers s on each asana—some easier, others more advanced, some using asana props: blankets, a cushion, a block, or a strap (see Appendix B: Further Exploration). If you have special needs because of a particular physical condition, a qualified teacher can help you find the variations that are best for you.

Keep a Straight Spine

Proper spinal alignment is essential for a successful yoga practice. Learn to feel whether your spine is straight (neutral, in its natural curves), and strive to keep it straight always, unless you're consciously bending it—or consciously *allowing* it to bend—as one does in certain asanas, for specific purposes. Just as a crimped garden hose impedes the flow of water, a significantly bent spine can impede the flow of energy to the brain. Paramhansa Yogananda often warned, "A bent spine is the enemy of Self-realization."

Use the Breath

Almost all asanas call for the breath to flow smoothly and easily, without strain. The belly should expand as you inhale, and relax back in as you exhale. Unless otherwise instructed, breathe through the nose and make your inhalations and exhalations equal in duration.

Breath and bodily movement will assist each other if, in general, you inhale as the body comes up and exhale when the body goes down. For example, inhale as you rise into Bhujangasana (Cobra Pose), and exhale as you exit. Exhale when going into Padahastasana (Hand-to-the-Foot Pose), and inhale as you exit. Chapter 4 notes a few exceptions to this guideline.

Connect with Energy

Although you can practice spiritual Hatha Yoga with no thought of energy, it's involved anyway. It's better to be able to work consciously with energy, both in your practice and in daily life. This begins with an *awareness* of energy. Chapter 1 offered several exercises to help you feel energy; here are several more:

- Try to feel the energy that flows out from your spine to move your body into an asana, activates your muscles as you hold the asana, and returns to the spine as you relax out of the asana. Use visualization to make those energy movements more real to you.
- Throughout your day, notice how your breath, your state of mind, and your emotional reactions are connected with upward or downward sensations in your torso; those sensations are movements of energy.
- Learn the Energization Exercises of Paramhansa Yogananda. They'll increase your energy, your awareness of it, and your ability to control it. The Energization system merits a study separate from the scope of this book, and I recommend it strongly (see Appendix B: Further Exploration).

Relax

Relaxation, both mental and physical, is just as important as mental and physical effort. Without relaxation, less energy will be available to you (it will be tied up as tension), and you'll lose your awareness and control of whatever energy *is* available to you; that will minimize the spiritual benefits of your practice. Here are some key points about relaxation:

- Relaxation doesn't mean to be lazy. No one slides downhill into divine bliss! Rather, try to relax in the midst of effort. In physically demanding asanas, foster relaxation by breathing slowly and smoothly, by releasing tension in body parts that don't need to be engaged, and by maintaining an attitude of calm enjoyment. Modify asanas as needed in order to have a sense of relaxation.
- When you reach your farthest point in a stretch, don't force your way past the resistance. Forcing might injure you, and it certainly lessens your awareness of energy. Instead, concentrate in the area of resistance and feel that your exhalations are dissolving the resistance so that you can relax farther into the stretch.
- Relaxation has a direction: most people relax downward, as when collapsing onto a couch. That won't raise awareness. Strive instead to relax inward and upward. For

example, as you exit an asana, visualize—and try to feel—energy releasing from your periphery, returning to your spine, then flowing upward toward your brain. It's easy to relax in this way; it's simply a shift of perspective. It's also spiritually beneficial, for inner awakening is a process, not of becoming something else, but of relaxing upward, away from preoccupation with that which you're not, and into what you've always been: divine bliss.

Engage with the Asana Affirmations

Each asana has one or more specific beneficial effects on your state of mind. As I mentioned in Chapter 1, bodily position alone can do only so much, but you can amplify its effects by using the power of your mind. One effective way to do so is unique to Ananda Yoga®: silently repeat a specially-crafted affirmation while holding the asana.

Each asana has its own affirmation that reinforces a particular positive effect of that bodily position on your state of mind. For example, Ardha Chandrasana (Half-Moon Pose; see photo) awakens a great deal of energy and stimulates subtle energy centers associated with attitudes of courage and steadfastness. As you hold the asana, amplify those effects by affirming silently,

"Strength and courage fill my body cells."

Mentally repeat the affirmation multiple times, with energy, willpower/willingness, and most important, with the quiet, confident *feeling* of strength and courage. Don't move your lips or tongue; just think the words and sensitively attune your mind to the qualities of strength and courage. This will help you go deeper into those qualities—ideally, go beyond the words of the affirmation into the pure feeling of those qualities. Different asanas strengthen different positive qualities, and therefore have different affirmations, but the affirmation *method* is always the same.

As with any new activity, it may take time before the asana affirmations feel natural in your practice. To speed the process—and to go deeper into the positive qualities—adopt the attitude of the affirmation as you first come into the asana. For example, don't wait for

Ardha Chandrasana or its affirmation to give you strength and courage; instead, practice the pose and affirmation *with* a strong, courageous attitude. That puts you on the wavelength of those qualities, so you can receive even more.

An Aid to Forward Bends

In Ananda Yoga, the primary purpose of forward-bending asanas is to open the astral spine so that energy can flow through it more freely. To accomplish this safely and effectively, it's helpful to practice forward bends in two phases: active and relaxation (see photos). In the active phase, focus on lengthening the spine and folding deeper in the hip joints, keeping the spine straight. This is excellent preparation for the full expression of the asana: the relaxation phase, in which you completely relax the lengthened spine into ever-greater openness (assuming that your spine is healthy and there's no discomfort in doing so). Although it's not essential to use two distinct phases, I've found it helpful in teaching as well as in my own practice, even after more than 30 years of experience. In Chapter 4, the instructions for forward bends address both phases.

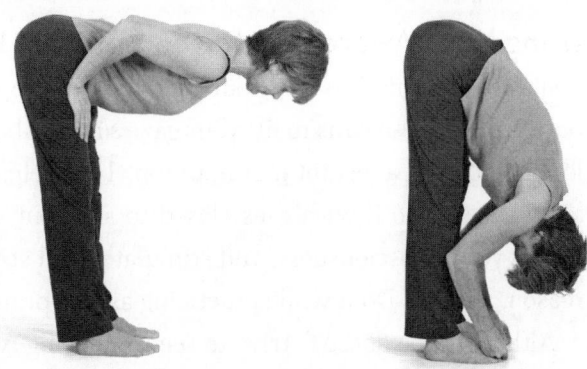

Active and relaxation phases of Padahastasana
(Hand-to-the-Foot Pose)

The final three principles of practice apply to pranayama and meditation as well as to asana. See Chapters 5 and 6 for additional principles specific to pranayama and meditation.

Aim High *and* Stay Grounded

In Ananda Yoga we practice with a feeling of lightness in the body, of lengthening upward through the body, and of lifting energy to the spiritual eye. Some people worry, however: "I'm already too disconnected from my body, and ungrounded. Won't lifting energy and feeling light make it worse?"

No, such people simply need to take some extra steps to stay grounded: Pay extra attention to all physical sensations. Breathe smoothly and easily, feeling the belly expand as you inhale, and relax back in as you exhale. Feel the connection between the floor and whatever parts of your body touch the floor; connect with that stability without *sinking* into it, without feeling heavy or passive. Relax also into your *inner* stability: into your center, into your sense of who you are, into your spine, into the present moment. It's also good to practice asanas that are particularly grounding, such as Vrikasana (Tree Pose), Virabhadrasana II (Warrior Pose II), Vajrasana (Firm Pose), Baddha Konasana (Bound Angle Pose), and Supta Vajrasana (Supine Firm Pose).

There's no conflict between being grounded and lifting your energy. Quite the contrary: both are essential for spiritual growth; blending the two simply requires a bit of practice for some people.

Bring Your Awareness to the Spiritual Eye

Yogis often counsel to "lift your gaze toward the spiritual eye" when you don't need to see outwardly. That means to lift your gaze *slightly* above horizontal, with relaxation, as though looking toward a distant mountaintop. This helps you gather energy and awareness at the spiritual eye; do it with eyes closed to shut out visual distractions, or with eyes open. It uplifts your consciousness, and stimulates and strengthens your concentration, willpower, reason, and joy. Do it while practicing asana, pranayama, meditation—and anytime.

Although one doesn't strive to see something when gazing toward the spiritual eye, you might see a subtle light if your mind is calm. And if your mind is *very* calm—as it becomes in deep meditation—you might see that light clearly as a golden ring surrounding a field of deep blue, in the center of which is a five-pointed, silvery-white star. This light is the spiritual eye. If you see it during asana practice, stop and sit down, then gaze intently yet calmly into that light, bathing yourself in its uplifting vibrations.

Be a Spiritual Artist

As much as possible during your practice, apply your "artistic faculties" (see Chapter 1): willpower, concentration, feeling, visualization, positive attitude, and devotion. It's not difficult, and discovering how to do it is part of the adventure: you, and only you, can make that discovery. Then, and only then, can your practice reach its full potential.

Above all, remember the faculty that empowers all the others: your spiritual aspiration, your devotion. Your heart wants something more, and that wanting is a precious resource. Bring devotion into your practice of all the techniques—not as a mere idea or wish, but as the heart's vibrant *feeling* of upward aspiration, yearning, and commitment. When you practice with devotion, in active partnership with Spirit, your energy will rise naturally, and your practice will become alive, uplifting, and deeply fulfilling.

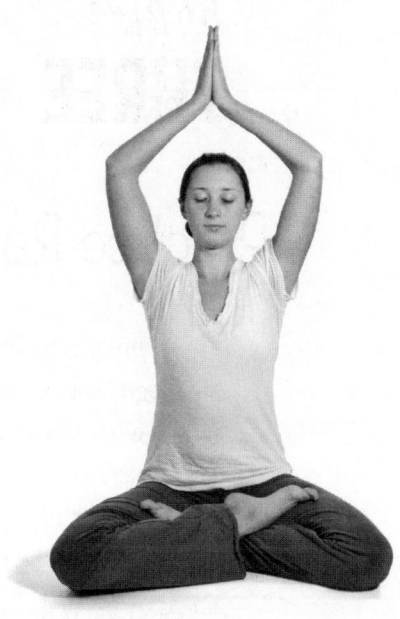

Chapter
THREE

Practice Routines

As you practice each pose, do not ask yourself merely, "What do the [yoga] books say I should be feeling in this position?" Feel, rather, what the total significance of the pose is to your own inner consciousness. As you move a hand, feel that your mind is moving with it. Feel, still more deeply, the relationship between outward movement and the inward movements of the soul.

—SWAMI KRIYANANDA

Now I'll show you how to weave asanas, pranayamas, and meditation into well-rounded Ananda Yoga® routines. Section 3.1 offers four sample routines that illustrate this approach, and Section 3.2 gives instructions for creating your own routines. First, a bit of terminology that will simplify those descriptions:

Active and Neutral Asanas

In a traditional Hatha Yoga practice such as Ananda Yoga, asanas are of two types:

- Active (requiring effort and/or stretch), and
- Neutral (requiring little or no effort or stretch)

Most asanas are active; hold them as long as you can stay concentrated and relaxed in the midst of effort—and, of course, as long as you're enjoying the experience. This gives you enough time to attune yourself with the state of mind that the bodily position naturally promotes.

Then exit to a neutral asana, and pause there to relax your awareness—and with it, the energy awakened by the preceding asana—into your center and upward toward the brain. When you've done as much of that as you can, and when you feel you've gained as much of the neutral asana's own special benefit as possible, move to the next active asana.

Naturally, most beginners will hold an active asana for a shorter time than will experienced practitioners: 15 seconds is a reasonable place to start, followed by a pause of 10–15 seconds in a neutral asana. For a deeper experience, gradually lengthen your time in the active asanas—and in the neutral asanas, too, if you can continue bringing energy inward and upward.

Remember: Neutral asanas are not mere resting positions to be eliminated if you're not tired. These pauses play a key role in bringing energy to the spiritual eye.[3]

3.1—SAMPLE ROUTINES

To understand the Ananda Yoga approach, I recommend that you explore some of the individual asanas (Chapter 4) and pranayamas (Chapter 5) in these routines before you practice. Even experienced practitioners might gain helpful insights by reading at least the opening paragraph of each technique; the page number is shown in parentheses after its English name.

Choose for yourself which sitting position(s) to use during pranayama practice at the beginning and end of each routine, as well as for meditation. See Chapter 6 for instruction in meditation.

Each routine calls for warm-up exercises, which I'll not describe here; you'll find a guided video warm-up sequence at AnandaYoga.org. Paramhansa Yogananda's Energization Exercises are ideal warm-ups, although their primary aim is much loftier (see Appendix B: Further Exploration).

To illustrate the interplay between active and neutral asanas, Routines 1 and 2 show neutral asanas in smaller, grey italic type below the name of each active asana. Because the neutral asanas to be practiced between the sides of a two-sided asana should be obvious, they're not shown. Insert neutral asanas similarly in Routines 3 and 4.

The approximate timings shown for Routines 1 and 2 are based on holding each active asana for about 15 seconds, then pausing in a neutral asana for 10–15 seconds. Timings for Routines 3 and 4 are based on holding each active asana for 25–30 seconds, and the neutral asanas for 10–15 seconds. For all four routines, hold the asanas even longer if you like—as long as you can breathe smoothly, stay relaxed in the midst of effort, and enjoy the experience. If you wish to add asanas to these routines, see the guidelines in Section 3.2.

---

[3] For a deeper exploration of the pauses, see my article "Playing the Pauses," online at AnandaYoga.org/pause.

Routine 1 (30 minutes)

For Beginners

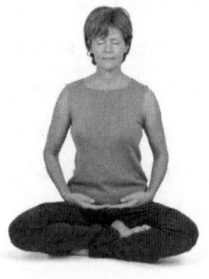

1 Dirgha Pranayama I
Full Yogic Breath
(page 154), 6 breaths

2 WARM-UP
EXERCISES
5 minutes

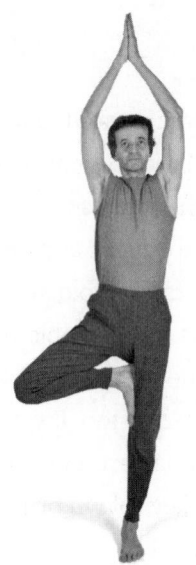

3 Vrikasana
Tree Pose (59)
Tadasana (58)

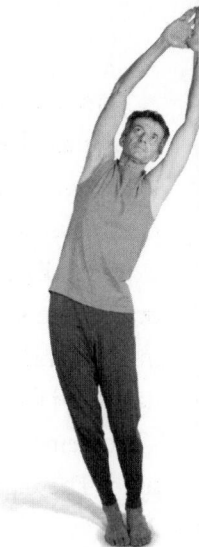

4 Ardha Chandrasan
Half-Moon Pose (7
Tadasana

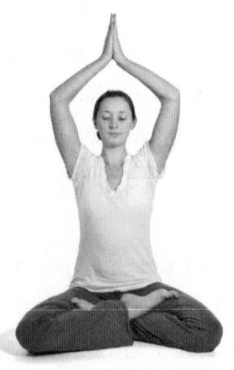

8 Parvatasana
(Seated) Mountain Pose (123)
Swastikasana

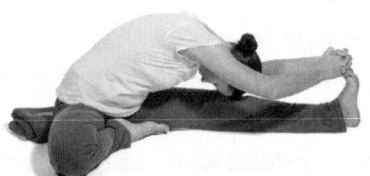

9 Janushirasana
Head-to-the-Knee Pose (84)
Swastikasana

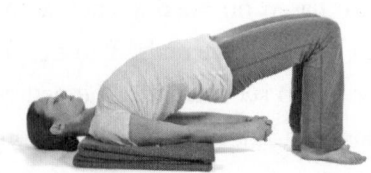

12 Setu Bandhasana
Bridge Pose (105)
Savasana

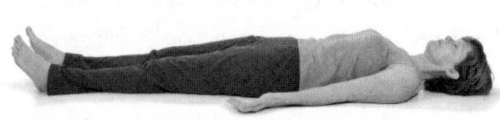

13 Deep Relaxation in Savasana
Corpse Pose (138), 3 minutes

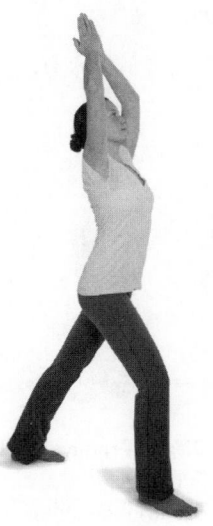

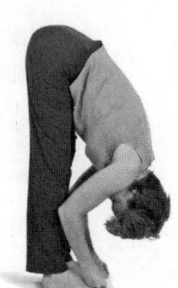

5 **Padahastasana**
Hand-to-the-Foot Pose (67)
Tadasana

6 **Muktasana**
Freedom Pose (72)
Tadasana

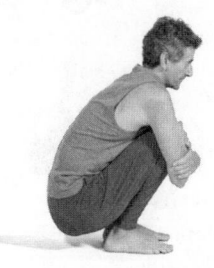

7 **Pavanamuktasana**
Wind-Freeing Pose (109)
Swastikasana (142)

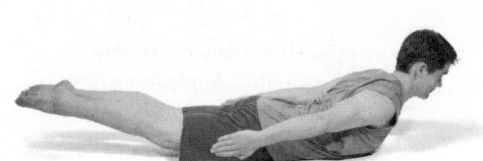

10 **Salabhasana**
Locust Pose (115)
Savasana (138)

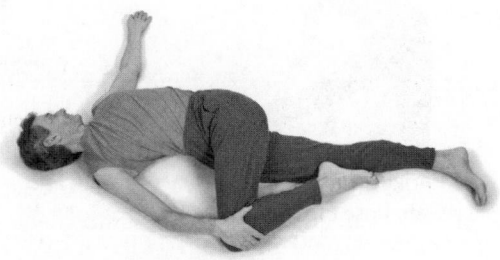

11 **Jathara Parivartanasana**
Supine Twist (99)
Savasana

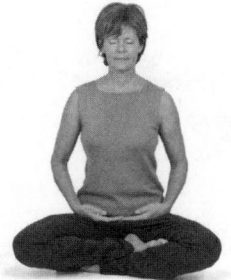

14 **Meditate**
for at least 5 minutes

Routine 2 (45 minutes)
For Beginners

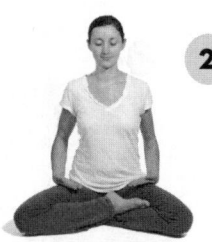

2 WARM-UP
EXERCISES,
5 minutes

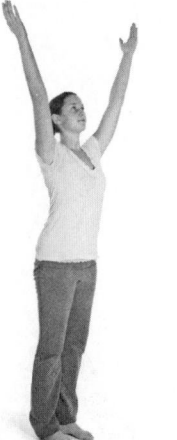

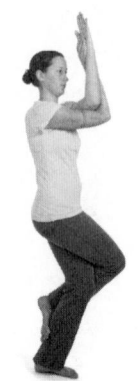

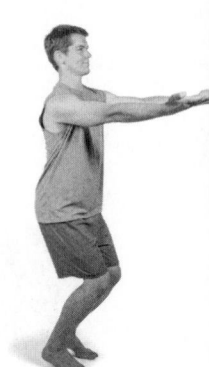

1 **Sitkari Pranayama**
Hissing Breath (page 158),
6 breaths
**Then concentrate at the
spiritual eye,**
6 breaths

3 **Dirgha Pranayama II**
Full Yogic
Breath Flow (155),
5 breaths
Tadasana (58)

4 **Garudasana**
Eagle Pose (60)
Tadasana

5 **Utkatasana**
Chair Pose (65)
Tadasana

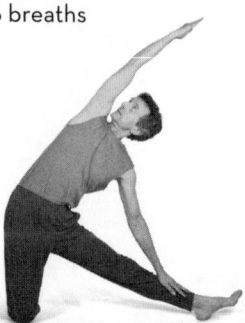

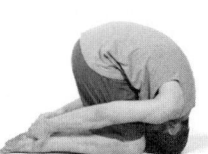

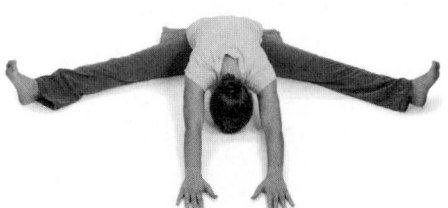

9 **Parighasana**
Gate Pose (96)
Vajrasana (143)

10 **Sasamgasana**
Hare Pose (91)
Balasana (137)

11 **Upavistha Konasana**
Seated Angle Pose (88)
Swastikasana (142)

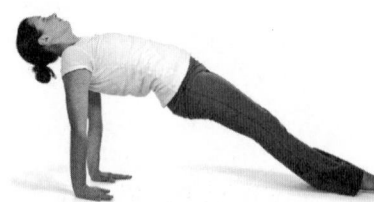

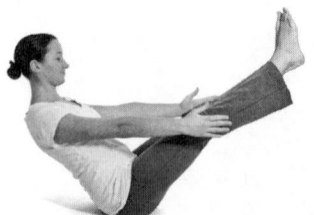

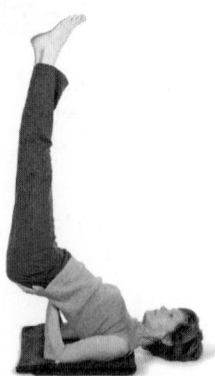

15 **Purvotanasana**
Front-Stretching Pose (114)
Swastikasana

16 **Navasana**
Boat Pose (112)
Swastikasana

17 **Viparita Karani**
Simple Inverted Pose (128)
Savasana (138)

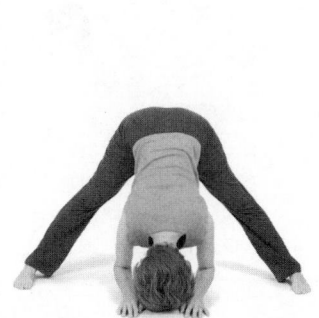

6 **Prasarita Padotanasana**
Wide-Stance Forward Bend (68)
Tadasana

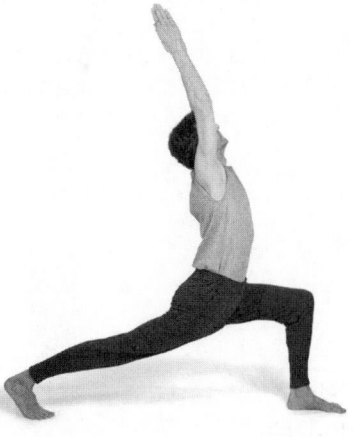

7 **Virabhadrasana I**
Warrior Pose I (74)
Tadasana

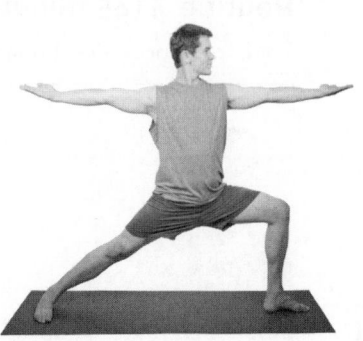

8 **Virabhadrasana II**
Warrior Pose II (75)
Tadasana

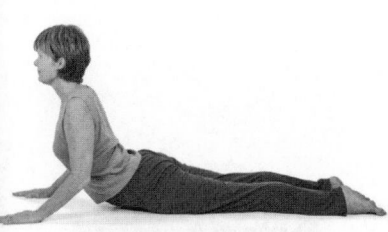

12 **Bhujangasana**
Cobra Pose (103)
Balasana

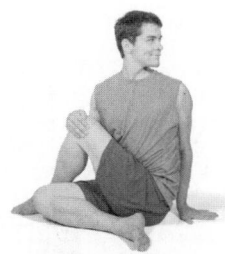

13 **Ardha Matsyendrasana**
Half Spinal Twist (97)
Swastikasana

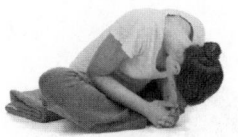

14 **Baddha Konasana**
Bound Angle Pose (87)
Swastikasana

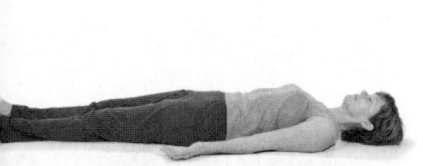

8 **Deep Relaxation in Savasana**
Corpse Pose (138), 5 minutes

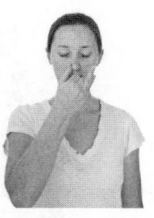

19 **Chandra Bheda Pranayama**
Expanding Moon Breath (161),
6–12 breaths

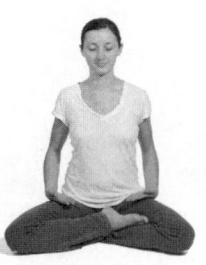

20 **Meditate for at least 5 minutes**

Routine 3 (45 minutes)

For Experienced Practitioners

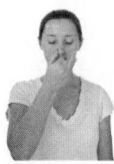

1 **Nadi Shodhanam**
Alternate Nostril
Breathing (page 163),
4 cycles (8 breaths)
**Then concentrate at
the spiritual eye,**
8 breaths

2 **WARM-UP
EXERCISES,**
5 minutes

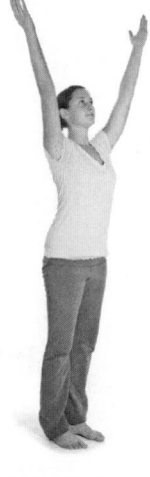

3 **Dirgha Pranayama II**
Full Yogic Breath
Flow (155), 5 breaths

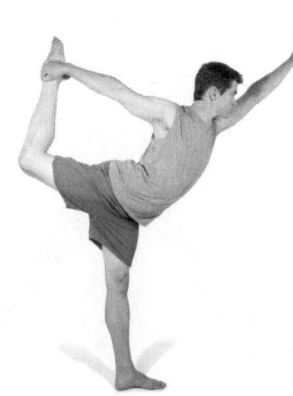

4 **Natarajasana**
King-of-the-
Dance Pose (61)

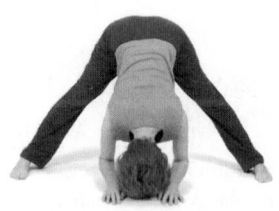

8 **Prasarita Padotanasana**
Wide-Stance Forward
Bend (68)

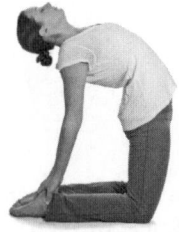

9 **Ustrasana**
Camel
Pose (100)

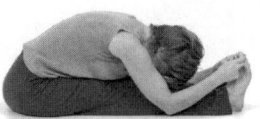

10 **Paschimotanasana**
Posterior-Stretching
Pose (85)

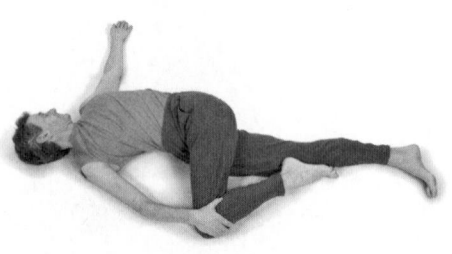

14 **Jathara Parivartanasana**
Supine Twist (99)

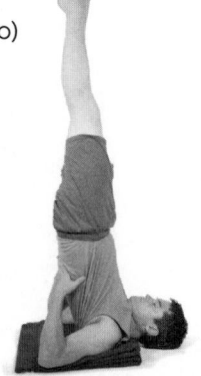

15 **Sarvangasana**
Shoulderstand (126)

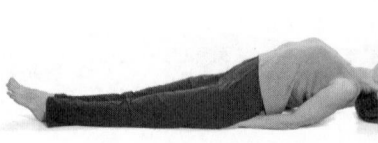

16 **Matsyasana**
Fish Pose (106)

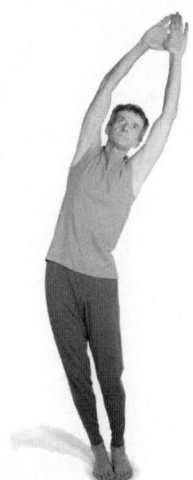

5 Ardha Chandrasana
Half-Moon Pose (71)

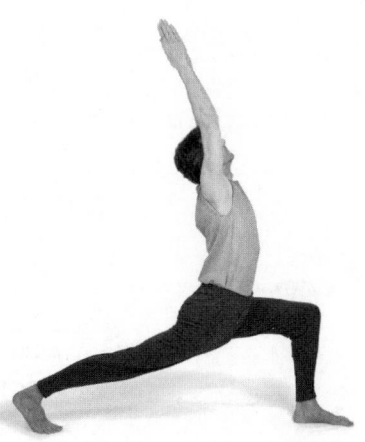

6 Virabhadrasana I
Warrior Pose I (74)

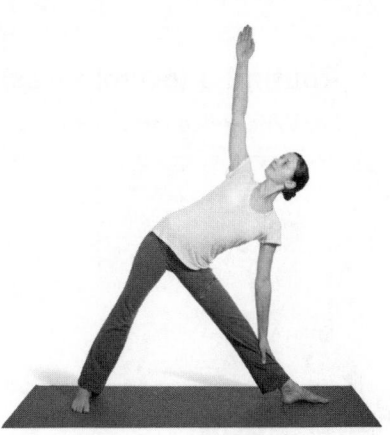

7 Trikonasana
Triangle Pose (76)

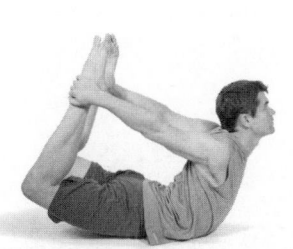

11 Dhanurasana
Bow Pose (117)

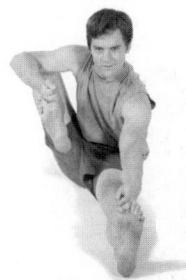

12 Akarshana Dhanurasana
Pulling-the-Bow Pose (113)

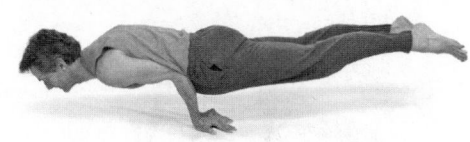

13 Mayurasana
Peacock Pose (119)

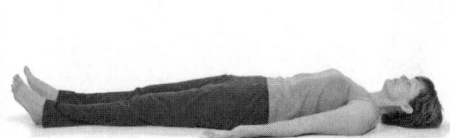

17 Deep Relaxation in Savasana
Corpse Pose (138),
3 minutes

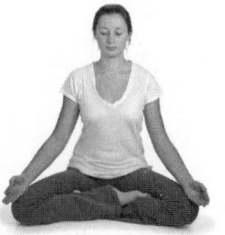

18 Ujjayi Pranayama with
Mula Bandha
Victorious Breath with Root
Lock (157, 165), 10 breaths

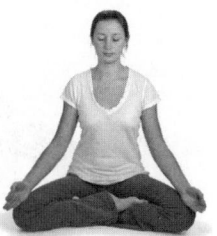

19 Meditate
for at least
10 minutes

Routine 4 (60 minutes)
For Experienced Practitioners

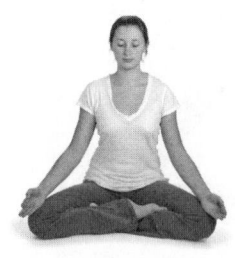

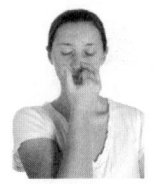

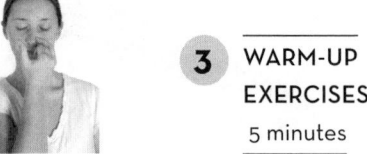

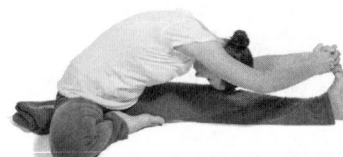

3 WARM-UP
EXERCISES,
5 minutes

1 **Dirgha Pranayama I**
Full Yogic Breath
(page 154), 6 breaths

2 **Surya Bheda Pranayama**
Expanding Sun Breath (162), 6 breaths
**Then concentrate at the
spiritual eye,** 8 breaths

4 **Surya Namaskar**
Sun Salutation (80)
3 cycles

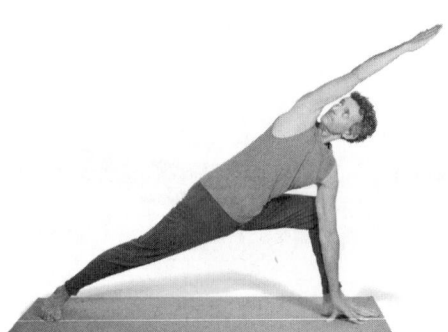

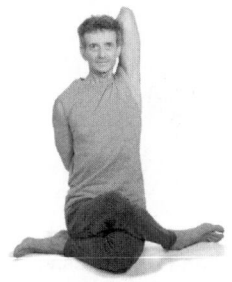

8 **Parsvakonasana**
Side Angle Pose (78)

9 **Gomukhasana**
Face-of-Light Pose (90)

10 **Janushirasana**
Head-to-the-
Knee Pose (84)

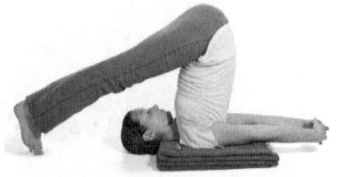

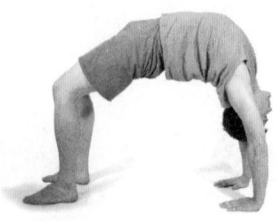

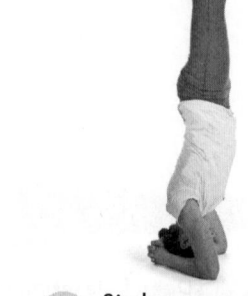

14 **Halasana**
Plow Pose (129)

15 **Chakrasana**
Wheel Pose (107)

16 **Sirshasana**
Headstand (132)

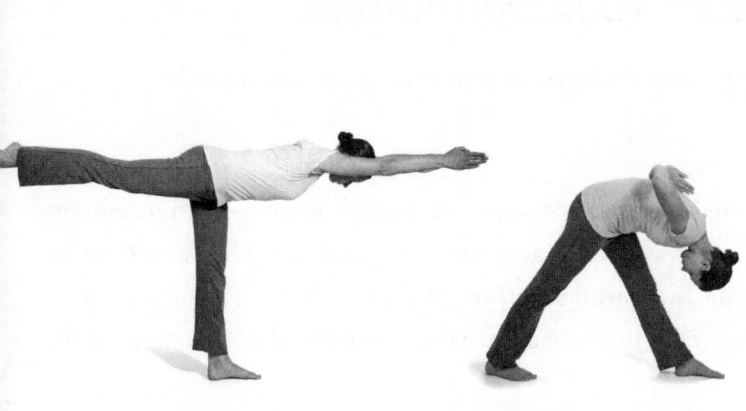

5 Ganapatiasana
Ganapati's Pose (62)

6 Parsvotanasana
Side-Stretching Pose (69)

7 Muktasana
Freedom Pose (72)

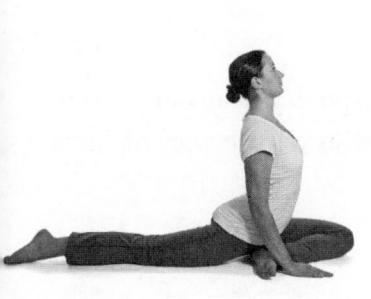

11 Rajakapotasana
Royal Pigeon Pose (102)

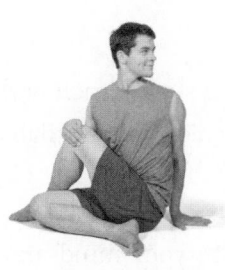

12 Ardha Matsyendrasana
Half Spinal Twist (97)

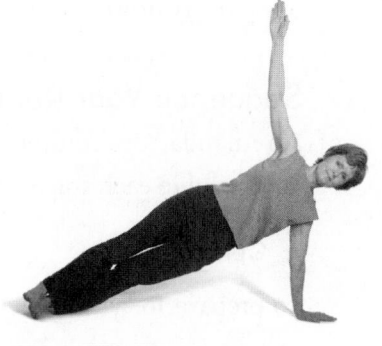

13 Vasishthasana
Vasishtha's Pose (118)

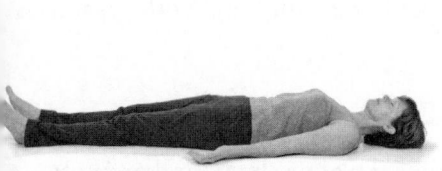

17 Deep Relaxation in Savasana
Corpse Pose (138), 5 minutes

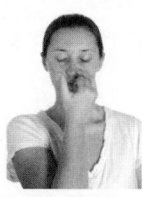

18 Surya Bheda Pranayama with
Jalandhara Bandha
Expanding Sun Breath with Chin
Lock (162, 166), 6–12 breaths

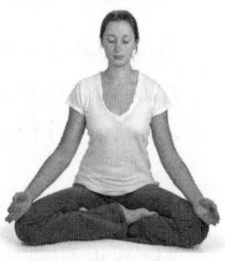

19 Meditate for at
least 10 minutes

3.2—CREATE YOUR OWN ROUTINE

Here are guidelines for creating routines tailored to your own goals and abilities:

Choose the Asanas

Include a balance pose, an inverted pose, and at least one of each basic spinal movement: forward bend, backward bend, sideways bend, and twist. Beyond this, choose according to your personal preferences, goals, and available time. If time is short, it's better to do a few postures slowly and well than to do many hastily. And, of course, always leave time for meditation.

The instructions in Chapter 4 suggest which neutral asana(s) might follow each active asana. It's simple: use neutral asanas that allow for natural transitions in your practice. Thus, after a standing asana, pause in Tadasana (Standing Mountain Pose). After a floor asana or inversion, you'll usually pause in a sitting asana, in Balasana (Child Pose), or in Savasana (Corpse Pose).

Sequence Your Routine

An Ananda Yoga routine has seven stages, each with its own purpose. The amount of time you spend in each stage will depend on your available time as well as your chosen emphasis.

1. Centering

To prepare for your practice, calm your mind and internalize your awareness by sitting upright and practicing one or two pranayama techniques. Then meditate for at least a few breaths, with eyes closed, gazing toward the spiritual eye.

2. Warm-Ups

Warm the muscles and joints to prepare the body to stretch safely. Harmonize your bodily movements with the breath to help you move more easily and gracefully, and with greater awareness of each movement.

3. Standing Asanas

These asanas help center your awareness in the spine, vitalize the entire body, and promote healthy posture.

4. Floor Asanas

After standing poses, go down on the floor for the following progression:

    a. Stretch and relax the extremities to withdraw energy from the periphery of the body into the spine.

    b. Next, stretch and open the physical spine to enable the astral spine to receive more energy, and to remove energy blockages in the astral spine.

    c. Finally, energize the opened spine: fill it with life-force, so that the inverted asanas can help you bring that life-force to the brain.

Practice stages 4a–4c more or less in the above order. Many asanas accomplish the aims of more than one of these stages, so keep in mind what you're trying to accomplish at each point in your practice.

5. Inverted Asanas

An inverted asana is one in which the spine is upside down, or nearly so. The greater the degree of inversion, the more the force of subtle gravity (see glossary) can help bring energy to the brain. If you don't feel to do a fully inverted asana (Section 4.5), use one or more partial inversions such as Sasamgasana (Hare Pose), Setu Bandhasana (Bridge Pose), or Adho Mukha Shvanasana (Downward-Facing Dog Pose).

6. Deep Relaxation in Savasana (Corpse Pose)

Stay in Savasana for up to 10 minutes—or even longer—in order to relax body and mind so completely that you transcend body awareness. Stay awake, though; Savasana is preparation for meditation, not for sleep!

If you feel to shorten the deep relaxation—not because you're restless, but because you're calm and centered, ready and eager to meditate—then follow that urge.

7. Meditation

Everything else in your routine, while enjoyable and beneficial, has set the stage for the highest, most powerful technique of Yoga: meditation (see Chapter 6). *Always* include it in your practice.

Chapter 4 organizes the asanas to correspond roughly to stages 3 through 7—"roughly" because many asanas could fit into more than one stage. For example, there are standing asanas that energize the spine (stages 3 and 4c) and inverted asanas that stretch and open the spine (stages 5 and 4b). Again, know what you're trying to accomplish at each point in your routine, and choose the asanas accordingly.

Balance Your Movements

The following two points aren't absolute rules; they're simply aids to a deeper practice:

First, when an asana moves you in one direction, move next in the opposite direction: forward bend, then backward bend; twist to the left, then twist to the right—always with a neutral asana between the two, of course. Such complimentary movements will help you bring your energy and awareness ever deeper into your center. In Ananda Yoga the ideal pairing of forward and backward bends usually has the forward bend first, then the backward bend. A forward bend opens the astral spine; the ensuing backward bend can then bring more energy into the spine, and that energy can flow more freely.

Second, in two-sided asanas (in which you move first one way, then the other), the left side of your body should have to work harder in the first half of the pose: in Trikonasana (Triangle Pose), stretch to the left first; in Garudasana (Eagle Pose), stand on the left leg first. Although it's not wrong to start with the right side—energy will still flow in the same fashion—the left-side-first approach can help you be more *aware* of energy[4]; the greater your awareness of energy, the more effectively you can work with it.

Include Pranayamas

Pranayamas (breathing exercises) help center your energy in the spine, bring energy to the brain, and calm the breath, heart, and mind. The two most natural times for pranayama practice are as the initial centering (stage 1) and after deep relaxation (stage 6), as a way to enter meditation. Other options include: after warm-ups (stage 2) to center your awareness in the spine before the standing asanas, or after standing asanas (stage 3) to center the energy awakened by those asanas.

Usually, the place for a longer pranayama practice is after deep relaxation; any earlier practice should usually be brief (say, 2–3 minutes) because, when practiced correctly for

---

[4] This point has subtle aspects that are beyond the scope of this book. In brief, the left-side-first approach harmonizes your physical activity with the natural flow of energy in the body as you breathe. Because you're in sync with that flow, it's easier to perceive and attune yourself with it.

a longer period, pranayama techniques will take you into such deep stillness that physical movement would be disruptive. Of course, if you're starting from a restless or agitated state, it may take more than a brief practice just to settle your mind enough to have a focused asana practice.

See Chapter 5 for more pranayama guidelines.

Include Meditation—Always

When time is tight, you may be tempted to skip meditation. And when, after all, is time *not* tight? Don't fall into this trap. If you truly want to raise your awareness, meditation is your most powerful tool. Use it.

Chapter
FOUR

Asanas

Every posture is associated with certain mental and spiritual states which, if you meditate on them while doing the posture, will come to you more easily than if you go through the postures absent-mindedly, or thinking only of their physical benefits.

—SWAMI KRIYANANDA

This chapter offers instructions for a broad spectrum of asanas. The main photo for each asana emphasizes some of the alignment points that are most important for both safety and a deeper experience.

The asanas are grouped in sections according to the guidelines for sequencing an Ananda Yoga® routine (as explained in Section 3.2). Please note that many asanas have multiple benefits, and would fit equally well in two or more sections. You'll find instructional video clips at AnandaYoga.org.

4.1—STANDING ASANAS:
CENTER YOUR AWARENESS IN THE SPINE

Tremendous joy and awareness are experienced as one's consciousness becomes centered sensitively in the spine. The spine is, indeed, the holy river of baptism in which the God-ward-moving soul becomes cleansed and regenerated in waters of divine joy.

—SWAMI KRIYANANDA

Standing asanas help you center your energy and awareness in the spine—in the astral spine especially. They also help you cultivate a *straight* physical spine, without which you can't relax properly while standing, nor can energy flow freely to the brain.

Being centered in your spine is important, not only for spiritual awakening, but for all daily activities: the more you remain centered in the spine, the more poised you'll be, ready to meet whatever comes your way. To this end, here are some points to keep in mind in standing asanas as well as anytime you're standing during normal daily activity:

Practice Tips

- Center your awareness in the astral spine, and make it the core of your experience. In active standing asanas, try to feel energy being sent from the spine to move the limbs or to hold a position. When you exit to Tadasana (Standing Mountain Pose), consciously relax that energy back into the spine, and up toward the brain.
- Lengthen upward through your entire body. Don't let your weight sink onto your feet; be stable, yes, but don't sink. That solid foundation is your launching pad; it enables you to lengthen upward and give body and mind a sense of vitality, lightness, and new possibilities.

Tadasana—(Standing) Mountain Pose

Starting your asana practice with Tadasana sets the tone for all the asanas by reinforcing inner stillness, sensitive listening, and willingness to offer yourself completely into your practice. Every time you return to Tadasana after an active standing asana, return also to that stillness, listening, and willingness. Express those qualities through your bodily posture, lift your gaze toward the spiritual eye, and listen inwardly for the silent guidance of your Higher Self, affirming,

"I stand ready to obey Thy least command."

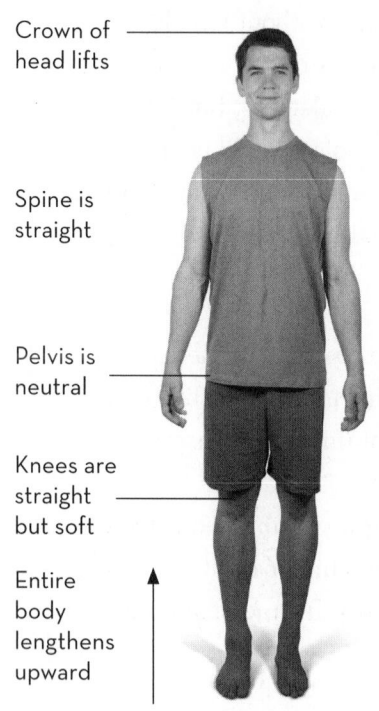

Crown of head lifts

Spine is straight

Pelvis is neutral

Knees are straight but soft

Entire body lengthens upward

Technique

Note: Proper standing posture (which Tadasana embodies) should feel light, balanced, stable, tall, supported, and above all, comfortable. Some postural habits, however, can make the alignment described below feel a bit uncomfortable. Don't try to correct everything all at once. Be patient and persistent, taking small steps toward proper posture, never rushing the process.

Stand with your feet hip-width apart, toes pointing forward. Tilt your pelvis forward or backward to establish the natural curves of your spine.

Place equal weight on both feet, and equal weight on the ball and heel of each foot. Lengthen up through your legs—with knees straight, neither bent nor locked—and up through your spine, all the way through the crown of your head. Relax your shoulders down away from your ears, and relax your arms and hands completely. Lift your gaze comfortably toward the point between the eyebrows (usually with eyes closed).

Ideally, viewed from the side, a vertical line through your ear canal would pass through the centers of your shoulder, hip, and knee joints, and just in front of your ankle. You can move toward this ideal over time; meanwhile, in the here and now, lift and open throughout your body to induce a feeling of lightness, alertness, and readiness.

Breathe smoothly and naturally, mentally affirming, *"I stand ready to obey Thy least command."*

Variation

• If it's difficult or uncomfortable to stand with your toes pointing directly forward, don't force it: let the toes turn out. If this difficulty is due to muscle imbalance, you may be able to correct it gradually by working with a qualified teacher. If it's due to joint structure, there may be no way to correct it, and that's okay: let your toes turn out.

Vrikasana—Tree Pose

Like all balance poses, this simple asana both requires and imparts a sense of centeredness in the spine. Keep your breath smooth and even, and feel a stabilizing current of energy flowing through your spine: upward with the inhalations, downward with the exhalations. Indeed, visualize that current flowing up and down through your entire body—from the standing leg all the way through your upward-pointing fingers. Affirm,

"I am calm, I am poised."

Shoulders and elbows relax

Spine is straight

Pelvis is neutral

Knee is straight (not locked)

Technique

Standing on your left foot, open your right hip so that your right knee swings out to the right. Your pelvis should face forward and stay level (not tipped sideways or tilted forward). Place the sole of your right foot on the inner left thigh, toes pointing down. Press foot and thigh against each other to help lengthen the spine, and lengthen upward through your left leg. To help you balance, fix your gaze on a point on the wall in front of you.

Inhale as you circle your hands out to the sides and overhead; join the palms, with fingers pointing upward. As you exhale, bend your elbows and soften your shoulders while keeping your spine long.

Breathe smoothly and naturally, silently affirming, *"I am calm, I am poised."*

Exit to Tadasana on an exhalation. Pause, then repeat on the other side.

Variations

- Easier: Leave the ball of your right foot on the floor and rest your right heel just above your left ankle.
- Easier: If tight shoulders prevent you from bringing your hands directly overhead without arching your spine, then either bend your elbows more, or join the palms at the heart.
- More advanced (half-lotus variation): Bring your right knee up near your chest, and hold the ankle with both hands. Flex the toes back toward the knee to stabilize the knee, then rotate your right hip joint to bring the knee out to your right; take care not to twist your knee. Place the right foot against the left leg at the hip crease, flex the toes toward the right knee stability, and press the little-toe side of the foot into your left thigh to prevent sickling (i.e., to keep the ankle from turning sideways significantly). Then join the palms overhead.

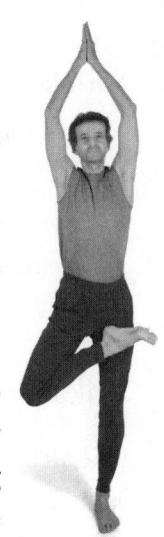

Garudasana—Eagle Pose (aka Twisted Pose)

Just as in your life, there's a lot going on in Garudasana. To keep from being distracted—in the asana and in your life—make the spine your point of focus. Experience the arms and legs as being wrapped around your spine, thereby accentuating your awareness of it. Feel that, though life may twist you in countless outward directions, inwardly you remain at peace, centered in your higher Self, as you affirm,

"At the center of life's storms, I stand serene."

Chest is lifted

Spine is straight and vertical

Neutral pelvis faces forward

Knee is slightly bent

Technique

Stand on your left foot, with your left knee slightly bent. Wrap your right leg in front and around the left leg as far as possible, keeping the pelvis facing forward and left thigh aligned with left toes. To help you balance, fix your gaze on a point on the wall in front of you.

Bring your left arm in front of you at the midline of your body, with the elbow bent 90 degrees and the forearm vertical. Wrap your right arm underneath and around your left arm, and join the palms, with fingers pointing upward. Keep your chest lifted, and your spine straight and vertical.

Breathe smoothly and naturally, mentally affirming, *"At the center of life's storms, I stand serene."*

To exit, release your arms, then inhale and reach them out to your sides. Exhale and relax into Tadasana. Pause, then repeat on the other side.

Variations

- Easier: If balance is difficult, rest your right toes on the floor to the outside of your left foot.
- Easier: If your palms won't come together, drape a strap between your left thumb and forefinger so that both ends of the strap hang down equally. Then wrap your right arm underneath and around the left arm as far as it will go, grasp the strap with your right hand, and gradually work your hands closer together along the strap.

Natarajasana—King-of-the-Dance Pose[5]

You can stay centered amid the fast pace and countless obligations of modern life if you make every action an *expansion* from your center, from your inner Self. Embody this principle in Natarajasana by reaching actively and equally from your center of gravity: back and up through the upraised leg, and forward and up through the spine and arm, affirming,

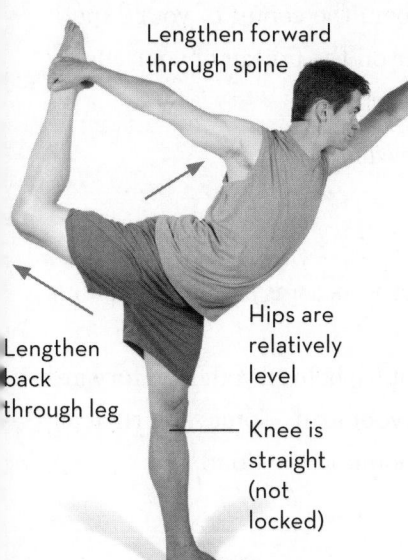

Lengthen forward through spine

Lengthen back through leg

Hips are relatively level

Knee is straight (not locked)

"While I move through life, I am anchored in my Self."

Technique

Stand on your left foot, bend your right knee, and grasp your outer right ankle with your right hand. Point the right knee toward the floor. To help you balance, fix your gaze on a point on the wall in front of you.

Inhale as you stretch your left arm overhead, then exhale as you bend forward from your left hip as far as balance and flexibility permit. Keep your left arm in line with your spine, and your left knee straight (not locked). Don't allow your right knee to drift out to the side.

Lengthen in opposite directions from your center of

---

5 To yogis, the dance is the divine dance of creation, preservation, and destruction—and the king of the dance is Shiva: the aspect of Spirit that dissolves creation back into Spirit.

gravity: forward and up through your spine and left arm, and backward and up through your right leg, as though trying to straighten the leg. This lengthening will draw you into a backward bend; tuck your pelvis as needed to prevent your lumbar spine from bending backward too far. The chest and pelvis may open a bit to your right; that's fine, but don't overdo it.

Breathe smoothly and naturally, silently affirming, *"While I move through life, I am anchored in my Self."*

To exit, inhale and return to upright, then exhale and release to Tadasana. Pause, then repeat on the other side.

Variation

• Grasp the inner right ankle instead of the outer. This variation helps keep the right knee from drifting out to the side and possibly twisting. However, it also requires substantial rotation of the right shoulder, so be careful not to strain your shoulder.

Ganapatiasana—Ganapati's[6] Pose

This asana brings a soaring sense of freedom—*if* you maintain a sense of fluidity, length, and grace. The breath can help you maintain those qualities: breathe smoothly and evenly, and feel/visualize the energy currents in the spine; make them the center of your experience. Try to embody the effortless flight of a bird as you soar on the breeze of your energy and aspirations, high above any self-limiting thoughts, affirming,

"I sail serenely through skies of inner freedom."

Technique

Stand on your left foot. On an inhalation, sweep your arms overhead, arms parallel and palms facing each other.

As you exhale, fold forward at the left hip and lift your right leg behind you. Fold forward as far as you can—all the way to horizontal if possible—with your arms, spine, and right leg in one straight line. To help you balance, fix your gaze on a point on the floor.

---

6   To yogis, Ganapati (aka Ganesha) symbolizes the endearing aspect of Spirit that helps one past the obstacles in one's life path.

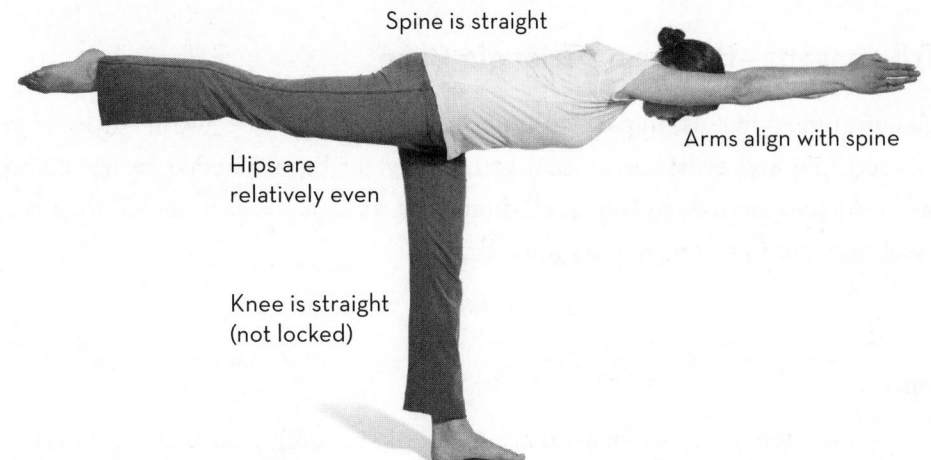

Spine is straight

Arms align with spine

Hips are relatively even

Knee is straight (not locked)

Keep your left knee straight (not locked), your right leg active, and the pelvis relatively square to the floor: don't lift its right side much, if at all. Lengthen equally in opposite directions: forward through the spine and arms, backward through the right leg.

Breathe smoothly and naturally, mentally affirming, "*I sail serenely through skies of inner freedom.*"

To exit, inhale and return to upright, then exhale and release to Tadasana. Pause, then repeat on the other side.

Variations

• Easier: Stretch your arms out to your sides, reaching in opposite directions.
• More advanced: Bring your palms together, fingers pointing forward and elbows straight but relaxed. Lift your head enough to gaze directly forward, just over your hands.

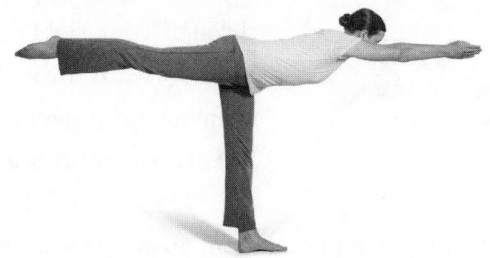

Tola Trikonasana—Balancing Triangle Pose

Expanded awareness means, in part, to experience life fully, to be aware—from your center—of everything and everyone around you. Cultivate that expanded awareness in Tola Trikonasana by lengthening *equally* in all directions, as though reaching out to experience the present moment in its entirety, as you affirm,

"I expand fully into this moment."

Technique

Stand on your left foot and fold forward at the left hip to bring your fingertips to the floor, with your spine straight. Lift the right leg behind you, into alignment with your spine; maintain this alignment throughout the asana.

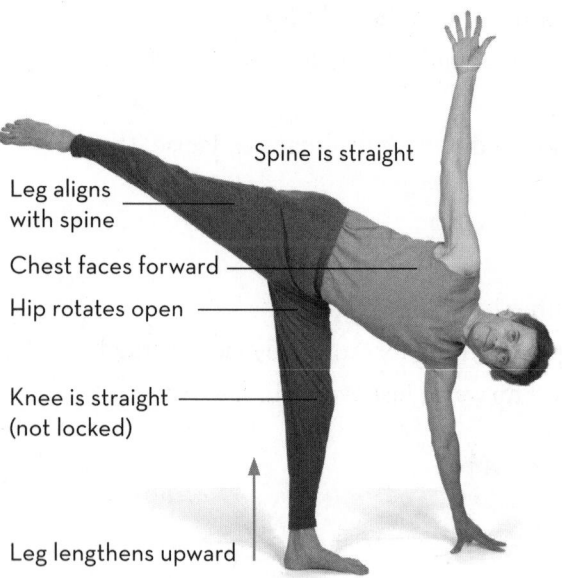

Spine is straight

Leg aligns
with spine

Chest faces forward

Hip rotates open

Knee is straight
(not locked)

Leg lengthens upward

On an inhalation, circle your right arm out to the right and up to vertical, rotating through your left hip joint to open your pelvis, chest, and head directly to the right. Keep your left knee straight (not locked). Use your left hand for stability, not to support weight. To help you balance, fix your gaze on a point on the wall in front of you.

Expand equally in all directions: down through your left arm and leg; up through your right arm; in opposite horizontal directions through your right leg and the crown of your head, forward through your chest and eyesight, even behind you with your intuitive perception. Breathe smoothly and naturally, silently affirming, *"I expand fully into this moment."*

To exit, bend your left knee; on an inhalation, push up with your left leg as you reach up with the right arm, and return to upright. Exhale into Tadasana. Pause, then repeat on the other side.

Variations

• Easier: Begin with your left foot parallel to, and a few inches away from, a wall. Enter the pose as above, but now with your back, left hip, and right foot resting against the wall.

• Easier: Stand with your back facing a wall before you enter the asana, close enough that your right foot will barely reach the wall once you enter. Once you have entered the asana, rest the toes lightly on the wall for stability.

• More advanced: Instead of gazing straight ahead, turn your head to gaze upward past your upraised arm. Be sure to keep your neck aligned with the rest of your spine.

Utkatasana—Chair Pose

As you hold Utkatasana, concentrate not on physical effort and endurance, but on the light-as-air *energy* reality of your body. The more you do so, the greater will be your sense of freedom from bondage to gravity's heavy, downward pull—not only on your body, but also on your energy and mind. You'll feel a sense of rising energy when you come out of the asana; savor it fully, and enjoy the accompanying lightness and ease. Affirm your freedom continually as you hold the asana, as well as after your exit:

"My body is no burden, it is light as air."

Technique

Standing in Tadasana, turn your palms forward. On an inhalation sweep your arms forward to horizontal, palms up, as you come up onto the balls of your feet. Retain your breath, and bend your knees as though sitting on the edge of a stool or high chair; lower your heels almost to the floor. Then exhale and breathe naturally, with shoulders relaxed. Your spine should be straight, and either vertical or tilted only slightly forward from the hips.

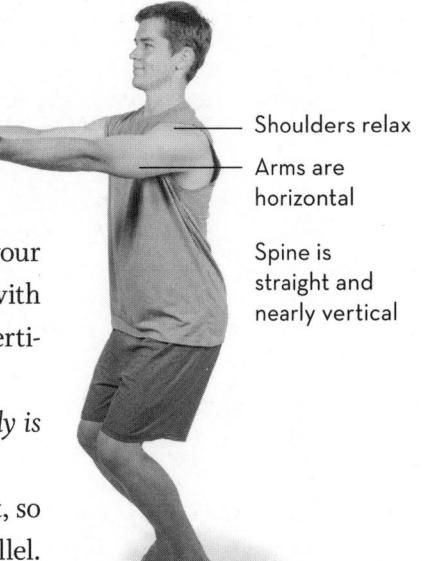

Shoulders relax

Arms are horizontal

Spine is straight and nearly vertical

Heels are lifted

Breathe smoothly and naturally, mentally affirming, *"My body is no burden, it is light as air."*

To enter the second phase of the pose, exhale into a full squat, so that your torso is vertical, and your thighs horizontal and parallel.

(Practice this phase only if you can enter it with control, and without straining your knees; see the variation below.) Place your hands on your thighs, palms up, where the thighs meet the abdomen; balance on the balls of your feet. Hold this position as long as comfortable, relaxing your legs and continuing the affirmation.

To exit, on an inhalation sweep your arms forward and up overhead as you come fully upright, then exhale into Tadasana and pause. You'll now feel a strong rush of energy from the legs into the torso. Use this experience of rising energy to increase your feeling of lightness of body and mind.

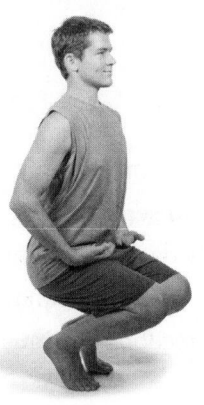

Variation

• Easier on the knees: In the second phase, a full squat—all the way down to the point where the legs can relax—puts considerable stress on the knees; even persons with healthy knees should be cautious, especially when coming up out of the squat. You can instead simply squat *farther* down than in the first phase—perhaps even quite far down, but not so far that you can relax the legs. The legs will have to work harder, but this variation gives more support to the knees, and it's even more energizing.

Padahastasana—Hand-to-the-Foot Pose (aka Jackknife Pose)

All forward bends open the astral spine; Padahastasana also partially inverts the spine so that energy can flow through that open spine toward the brain. On another level, the inverted position of the upper body contrasts with the upright position of the lower body, disrupting your customary sense of bodily heaviness: your lower body is as heavy as usual, but your upper body seems to have no weight at all. Accentuate this contrast energetically: actively lengthen up through the legs and release down through the spine. These contrasts bring a sense of freedom from gravity and from all heaviness. Deepen that feeling of freedom by affirming silently,

"Nothing on earth can hold me!"

Technique

From Tadasana, inhale as you stretch your arms overhead to lengthen your spine. As you exhale, circle your arms out to the sides and fold forward from your hips as far as possible without rounding your spine. Rest your hands on your thighs, just below the hip joints.

Active phase: Continue in this position for several breaths. On each inhalation, press your hands into the thighs and lengthen your spine. On each exhalation, fold a bit more at the hip joints, spine still straight. Actively lengthen up through your legs, keeping your knees straight (not locked).

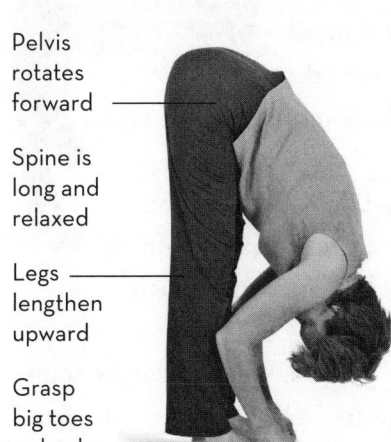

Pelvis
rotates
forward

Spine is
long and
relaxed

Legs
lengthen
upward

Grasp
big toes
or backs
of legs

Relaxation phase: When you've folded forward as far as possible with a straight spine, lengthen your spine with one last inhalation, then exhale and relax into the completed asana. Let gravity lengthen your spine and draw the crown of your head toward the floor; let your spine round if it's healthy and there's no discomfort. Wrap the first two fingers of each hand around the corresponding big toe, but don't pull yourself farther down. Go deeper into the forward bend only through relaxation, not through effort.

Breathe smoothly and naturally, silently affirming, *"Nothing on earth can hold me!"*

To exit, bend your knees and straighten your spine. Then with an inhalation, press down with your feet and return to upright as you circle your hands out to the sides and overhead; stretch tall. Exhale as you relax your arms down. Pause in Tadasana.

Variations

• Easier: Instead of reaching for the toes, lightly grasp the backs of your thighs, calves, or ankles, wherever you can reach easily. Whatever you grasp, don't pull on it to force yourself into a deeper forward bend. Rather, use it as a point of stability and support, so you can relax more deeply.

• Easier: Bend your knees to relieve any lower back discomfort, or if only with bent knees can you achieve any spinal inversion at all in the relaxation phase.

Prasarita Padotanasana—Wide-Stance Forward Bend

Standing forward bends foster freedom from the sense of physical and mental heaviness. The wide position of the feet in this one adds a sense of openness—of the spine, of the breath, and especially of the mind. Hold your mind open to the energy cascading through the spine to the brain, washing away mental tensions, worries, and regrets as you affirm,

"I relax and cast aside all mental burdens."

Technique

Step your feet wide apart. Inhale as you stretch your arms overhead to lengthen your spine. As you exhale, circle your arms out to the sides and fold forward from your hips as far as possible without rounding your spine. Rest your hands on your thighs, just below the hip joints.

Active phase: Continue in this position for several breaths. On each inhalation, press your hands into the thighs and lengthen your spine. On each exhalation, fold a bit more at the hip joints, spine still straight. Actively lengthen up through your legs, keeping your knees straight (not locked).

Relaxation phase: When you've folded forward as far as possible with a straight spine, lengthen your spine with one last inhalation, then exhale and relax into the completed asana. Let gravity lengthen your spine and draw the crown of your head toward the floor; let your spine round if it's healthy and there's no discomfort. Place your hands on the floor

Spine is long and relaxed

Pelvis rotates forward

Lengthen up through legs

Crown of head releases toward floor

beneath your shoulders. Go deeper into the forward bend only through relaxation, not through effort. Breathe smoothly and naturally, silently affirming, *"I relax and cast aside all mental burdens."*

To exit, bend your knees and straighten your spine. Then, on an inhalation, press down with your feet and return to upright as you circle your hands out to the sides and overhead; stretch tall. Exhale as you relax your arms down and step your feet back together. Pause in Tadasana.

Variations

- Easier: Bend your knees to relieve any lower back discomfort, or if only with bent knees can you achieve any spinal inversion at all in the relaxation phase.
- More advanced: Grasp your ankles instead of placing the hands on the floor.

Parsvotanasana—Side Stretching Pose (aka Pyramid Pose)

This asana expresses—and promotes—surrender of the small self and all its limitations, into divine grace. With the arms behind, the chest opens and the body can better express the spirit of willing surrender. The simple yet powerful hand mudra, aided by the pull of subtle gravity, directs energy through the medulla (the seat of ego) toward the brain. Keep your spine long and open in order to experience this self-offering on ever-deeper levels:

"I offer myself fully into the flow of grace."

Technique

From Tadasana, step your right foot back about 3 feet, and turn it out just enough that the heel rests on the floor and you're stable. Square your pelvis unless your right foot is turned out so much that doing so would twist the right knee. Join your palms behind you, fingers pointing upward along the spine.

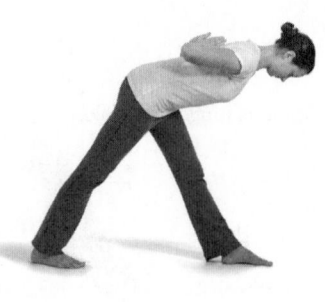

Active phase: On an inhalation, lengthen your spine, then exhale and fold forward from the hips, over the left leg, as far as you can with a straight spine. The left knee is straight (not locked). Press the ball of the left foot into the floor to distribute your weight as evenly as possible on both legs. Lengthen your straight spine with each inhalation, and fold forward a bit more with each exhalation.

Spine is long and relaxed

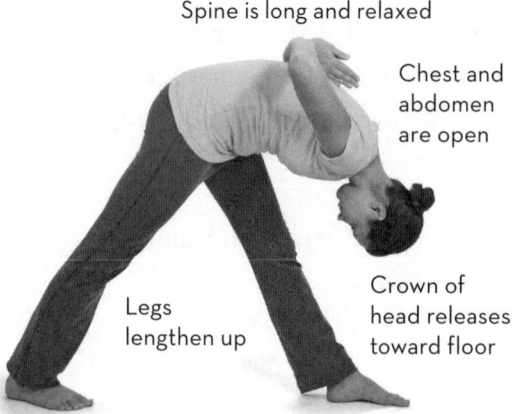

Chest and abdomen are open

Legs lengthen up

Crown of head releases toward floor

Relaxation phase: When you've folded forward as far as possible with a straight spine, lengthen your spine with one last inhalation, then exhale and relax into the completed asana. Let gravity lengthen your spine and draw the crown of your head toward the floor; let your spine round if it's healthy and there's no discomfort. Go deeper into the forward bend only through relaxation, not through effort. Feel the energy of your hands and fingers, aided by subtle gravity, directing energy through the spine to free the ego-centered energy of the medulla and carry it toward the spiritual eye.

Breathe smoothly and naturally, mentally affirming, "*I offer myself fully into the flow of grace.*"

To exit, bend your left knee and straighten your spine. Release your hands and, with an inhalation, sweep the arms overhead as you step the right foot forward beside the left. Exhale into Tadasana. Pause, then repeat on the other side.

Variations

- Easier: If you're unable to join your palms behind you, then join your palms at the heart.
- Easier: If balance is difficult, you can instead rest your hands on the left thigh near the hip joint. You can also step the right foot farther out to the side.

Ardha Chandrasana—Half-Moon Pose

To realize the full energizing potential of this pose, create the crescent-moon shape with your entire body, not just with your spine and arms. Don't bend so far to the side that you inhibit your breathing, as that would also inhibit the flow of energy in the spine. With energy flowing freely through the graceful arc of your body, you'll feel a powerful lifting sensation—especially in the legs and spine. Align your will with that lifting sensation as you affirm,

"Strength and courage fill my body cells."

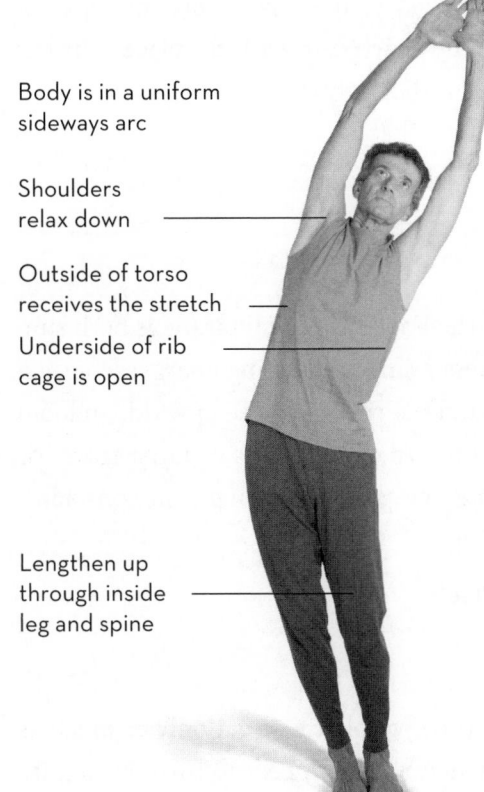

Body is in a uniform sideways arc

Shoulders relax down

Outside of torso receives the stretch

Underside of rib cage is open

Lengthen up through inside leg and spine

Technique

Stand with your feet together, arms at your sides, palms facing forward. On an inhalation, circle your hands out to the sides and up, rising onto the balls of your feet. Interlock your thumbs overhead, palms facing forward, and stretch tall. As you exhale, extend the stretch to the left with your upper body, and slide your hips to the right, heels slightly off the floor (or lightly touching the floor if needed). Fold to the left in the left hip joint, so that the right hip is higher than the left; don't let your weight sink into either hip.

The entire body now forms a graceful sideways arc. Stretch your body upward just as much as to the side; don't bend so far to the side that your breathing is inhibited. Actively lengthen up and to the left through the entire left side of your body (shoulders relaxed away from ears), thereby lifting and opening the right side to receive greater vitality; let the right heel lift if it does so naturally. Align your neck with the sideways arc of the rest of your spine, and without twisting your neck, gaze upward toward the spiritual eye.

Keep your body in a single plane, as though pressed between two panes of glass—not

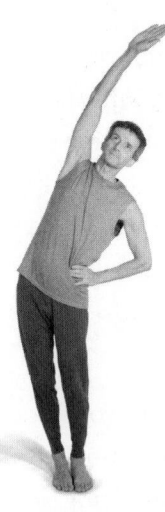

twisting, leaning forward, or arching backward. Tuck your pelvis if needed to keep your lumbar spine neutral.

Breathe smoothly and naturally, silently affirming, *"Strength and courage fill my body cells."*

To exit, inhale and stretch upright, then exhale as you circle your hands back to Tadasana. Pause, then repeat on the other side.

Variations

• Easier: If tight shoulders prevent you from bringing your hands directly over-head without arching your spine, then bend your elbows more, or separate your hands, or simply join the palms at the heart. Alternatively, place your left hand on the upper left rim of the pelvis, so that only the right arm is overhead, palm facing forward.

Muktasana—Freedom Pose

A natural choice to follow Padahastasana (Hand-to-the-Foot Pose), Muktasana is both simple and subtle. The key is to use your body to express rising, expanding energy: lengthen upward through the back leg, lift the chest and expand the rib cage, gaze upward, and join the palms with fingers pointing upward. Begin this upward expansion as you first enter the asana: sweep your arms forward and upward, feeling that you're sweeping your consciousness upward in triumphant, joyful freedom, affirming,

"I am free! I am free!"

Technique

From Tadasana, step your left foot back 2½–3 feet. Turn your left foot out only as much as needed for balance. Face your pelvis forward unless your left foot needs to turn out significantly, in which case allow your pelvis to open slightly to the left, so that you don't twist the left knee. Bend your right knee so that it's directly over your right ankle. Throughout this asana, keep equal weight on both feet.

With your lower body stationary, inhale as you sweep your arms forward and overhead, lifting your heart and drawing the upper spine into a backward bend. Join your palms, fingers pointing upward. As you exhale, relax your shoulders down and bend your elbows slightly, but don't sag

Shoulders and
elbows relax

Chest lifts

Spine is in
a uniform
backward arc

Lengthen up
through leg

Distribute weight
evenly on both feet

backward; keep equal weight on both feet. Arch the neck back in the same graceful backward arc as the rest of the spine, and gaze upward.

The backward bend of your spine may look slight, but it shouldn't *feel* slight: draw the bend strongly into the area behind the heart, and let the front and sides of your rib cage expand. Tuck your pelvis as needed to prevent your lumbar spine from bending backward too far.

Feel your entire body—from the upward thrusting back leg to the upward pointing fingers overhead—helping to lift energy up through the body. Breathe smoothly and naturally, mentally affirming, *"I am free! I am free!"*

To exit, inhale and reach up as you step forward with your left foot, then exhale into Tadasana. Pause, then repeat on the other side.

Variation

• Easier: If tight shoulders prevent you from bringing your hands directly overhead without overarching your spine, then bend your elbows more, or join the palms at the heart.

Virabhadrasana I—Warrior Pose I

This is the "horizontal cousin" of Muktasana (Freedom Pose). While the latter expresses rising into superconscious freedom—beyond the confines of body, personality, likes and dislikes, and limiting self-concepts—Virabhadrasana I emphasizes another necessity: aligning human will with divine will in order to do what one needs to do in this world. Feel as though you're offering your human will into divine will, that you be guided rightly in all that you do. Affirm,

"I attune my will to the Source of all power."

Technique

Shoulders relax

Spine is in a slight, uniform backward bend

Back of leg lifts

Knee directly above ankle

Thighs and toes align

Step your feet wide apart. Pivot 90 degrees to your left, keeping the right leg straight, and allowing the right heel to come off the floor, pointing straight behind you. Square your hips.

Bend your left knee into a deep lunge. Bring your thigh as close to horizontal as possible, and make sure it points in the same direction as the toes. Widen or narrow your stance so that the left knee is directly over the ankle. Lift strongly through the back of the right thigh.

On an inhalation, sweep your arms forward and up overhead, lifting your chest and your gaze, so that you come into a backward bend. Don't sag backward or bend your neck back sharply; rather, lift up strongly through the spine—especially through the heart area—and tuck your pelvis as needed to prevent your lumbar spine from bending backward too far. Your palms are apart and facing each other; your shoulders are relaxed.

Breathe smoothly and naturally, silently affirming, *"I attune my will to the Source of all power."*

To exit, inhale as you straighten your left leg, reach up, and turn to face forward once again. Exhale and relax your arms to your sides. Pause in this wide-stance position, then repeat on the other side.

Variation

• Instead of pointing the right heel behind you, keep the entire sole of the foot on the floor and let the right hip trail the left hip enough that you don't twist the right knee. This variation makes it easier to balance, but demands more hip flexibility; you might also find that it offers less upward opening.

Virabhadrasana II—Warrior Pose II

This is a particularly natural asana in which to transcend physical effort, and let divine energy do the pose *through* you. The upturned palms help you to be more receptive to divine energy. As you deepen the lunge, you'll free up even more energy. Your time in the asana—and the amount of energy flowing through you—is limited only by the span of your willing and joyful concentration on that energy. Feel that energy as being more real than your physical body; concentrate deeply on the energy as you affirm,

"I joyfully manifest the power of God!"

Technique

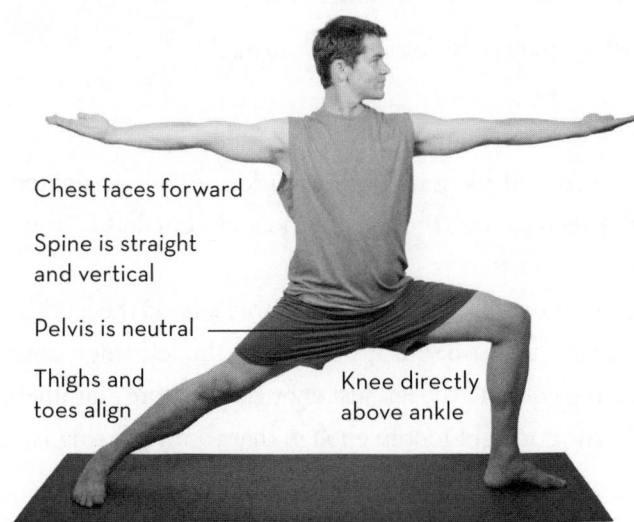

Chest faces forward

Spine is straight and vertical

Pelvis is neutral

Thighs and toes align

Knee directly above ankle

Step your feet wide apart. Pivoting from the left hip joint, turn your left leg out 90 degrees. Bend your left knee into a sideways lunge. Bring the thigh as close to horizontal as possible, and widen or narrow your stance so that the left knee is directly over the ankle. Place your feet so that a line from the second toe through the heel of your left foot will intersect the middle of the instep of your right foot.

Your left thigh should point in the same direction as the left toes. Ideally, the pelvis should face forward, but if that brings the left thigh out of alignment with the left toes, then rotate the pelvis to the left just enough to restore alignment; your chest continues to face forward. Turn your right foot in enough that your right thigh and right toes also align with each other.

Face your chest forward, with your hips level and spine neutral (you may need to tuck your pelvis to keep your lumbar spine neutral). Stretch your arms out to your sides, with palms facing up and shoulders relaxed. (Downturned palms affirm self-sufficiency rather than Self-sufficiency.) Rotate your head to gaze past your extended left arm.

Breathe smoothly and naturally, mentally affirming, *"I joyfully manifest the power of God!"*

To exit, inhale as you straighten your left leg and turn to face forward once again. Exhale and relax your arms to your sides. Pause in this wide-stance position, then repeat on the other side.

Trikonasana—Triangle Pose

Trikonasana helps you cultivate vibrant openness, vitality, and joy—all of which depend upon the free and abundant flow of the spinal energies. To promote that flow, keep the spine relatively straight; bending too much to the side inhibits the flow. This means not touching the floor with your hand if flexibility doesn't easily take it there; touching the floor is not the point of Triangle Pose. The truly important emphases are length, openness, and vitality, so that you can *experience*, not merely repeat, the affirmation,

"Energy and joy flood my body cells! Joy descends to me!"

Technique

Step your feet wide apart. Pivoting from the left hip joint, turn your left leg out 90 degrees. Place your feet so that a line from the second toe through the heel of your left foot will intersect the middle of the instep of your right foot.

Your left thigh should point in the same direction as the left toes. (Briefly bend the left knee to check this.) Ideally, the pelvis should face forward, but if that brings the left thigh out of alignment with the left toes, then rotate the pelvis to the left just enough to restore alignment; your chest continues to face forward. Turn your right foot in enough that your right thigh and right toes also align with each other.

Lift your left kneecap by slightly contracting the left thigh, thereby stabilizing the knee. Reach your arms out to your sides. On an inhalation, stretch your torso and left arm to your left and slightly upward, while you fold deeply in your left hip joint.

When you've stretched and folded as far as possible, exhale and rest your left hand lightly on your left leg or the floor, wherever it reaches easily. Keep your chest facing forward and your spine relatively straight, so the underside of your rib cage stays open. Don't rest substantial weight on the left hand; then you'll feel the most energy and joy in Trikonasana.

Raise your right arm to vertical, palm facing forward. Relax your shoulders down away from your ears. Lengthen your neck and keep it aligned with the rest of the spine as you rotate your head to look up past your right hand.

Breathe smoothly and naturally, mentally affirming, *"Energy and joy flood my body cells! Joy descends to me!"*

To exit, rotate your head to look forward. Bend your left knee, and as you inhale, press down with your left foot and reach up through your right hand to come upright, turning the toes forward. As you exhale, relax your arms to your sides. Pause in this wide-stance position, then repeat on the other side.

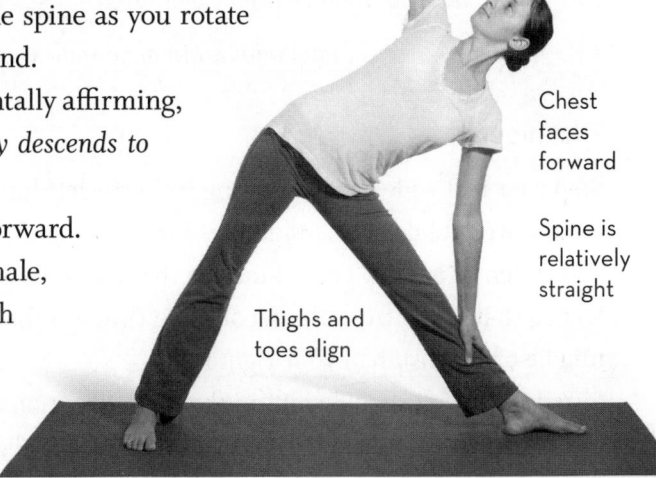

Neck rotates evenly

Chest faces forward

Spine is relatively straight

Thighs and toes align

Variations

• More advanced: The asana can be even more energizing—and more challenging—if, instead of resting your left hand lightly on the left leg, you hover the hand slightly in front of the leg, palm facing forward.

• More advanced: As you enter the asana, reach your torso not only to the side, but somewhat forward, almost to 45 degrees. Your left hand will thus have to reach back somewhat to touch the left leg. Open your chest and shoulders by bringing the right shoulder blade back, and the left shoulder blade forward; this adds a spinal twist to the standard asana. Because the chest needs to stay open, most people will find it best not to bring the torso as far down as in the standard asana. For safe knee alignment, turn the left foot out at an angle closer to 45 degrees than to 90 degrees.

Parsvakonasana—Side Angle Pose

Openness, length, and a good bit of lift bring forth the power of Side Angle Pose. To foster these qualities, keep your chest facing forward and your spine straight, in line with your upper arm and back leg. Never collapse your weight onto your lower arm; rather make your legs do most of the work of holding you up. Focus on the abundant energy flowing through your entire body as you breathe. Celebrate that strength and vitality, affirming,

"I am a fountain of boundless energy and power!"

Technique

Step your feet wide apart. Pivoting from the left hip joint, turn your left leg out 90 degrees. Bend your left knee into a sideways lunge. Bring the thigh as close to horizontal as possible, and widen or narrow your stance so that the left knee is directly over the ankle. Place your feet so that a line from the second toe through the heel of your left foot will intersect the middle of the instep of your right foot.

Your left thigh should point in the same direction as the left toes. Ideally, the pelvis should face forward, but if that brings the left thigh out of alignment with the left toes, then rotate the pelvis to the left just enough to restore alignment; your chest continues to face forward. Turn your right foot in enough that your right thigh and right toes also align with each other.

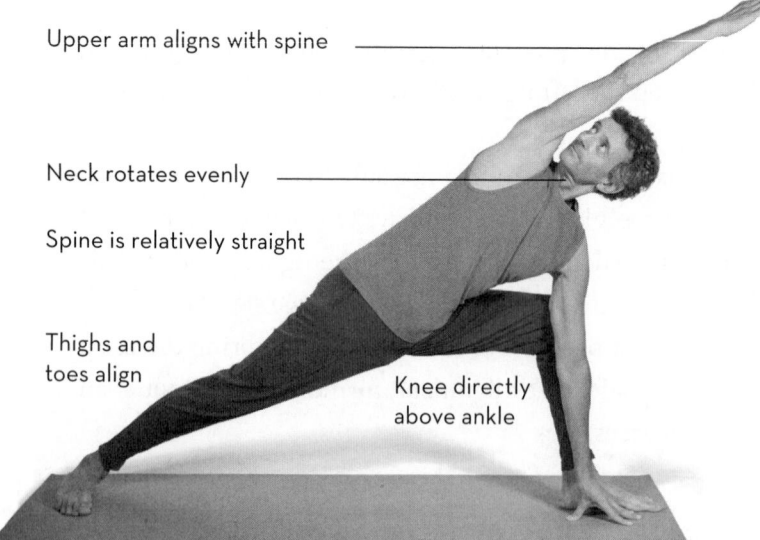

Upper arm aligns with spine

Neck rotates evenly

Spine is relatively straight

Thighs and toes align

Knee directly above ankle

Reach your arms out to your sides. On an inhalation, stretch your torso and left arm to your left and slightly upward, while you fold deeply in your left hip joint.

When you've stretched and folded to the left as far as possible, exhale and place your left hand *lightly* on the floor by your left instep. Keep your spine relatively straight, so the underside of your rib cage stays open. Face your chest forward. Circle your right arm up and over, in line with your spine and right leg; relax the right shoulder away from your ear, and turn the palm toward the floor.

Lengthen your neck and keep it aligned with the rest of the spine as you rotate your head to look up past your right upper arm. Don't look up at your right hand, as that would bring your neck out of alignment with the rest of your spine.

Breathe smoothly and naturally, silently affirming, *"I am a fountain of boundless energy and power!"*

To exit, rotate your head to look forward. As you inhale, press down with your left foot and reach up through your right hand to come upright, turning the toes forward. As you exhale, relax your arms to your sides. Pause in this wide-stance position, then repeat on the other side.

Variations

• Easier: Instead of bringing your left hand to the floor, rest your left elbow on your left thigh. Keep both legs engaged and don't rest substantial weight on your left thigh; relax your left shoulder away from your left ear. Most people will find that this variation is the only way they can keep a straight spine in Parsvakonasana—and that's fine, because it's the abundant flow of energy that's important; touching the floor isn't.

• More advanced: Place your left hand to the outside of the left foot. As you hold the asana, press the left knee into the left arm to help you open the left hip and the torso. Practice this variation only if you can keep your spine straight, chest facing forward, and left thigh still aligned with left toes.

Surya Namaskar—Sun Salutation

This sequence of asanas is vitalizing, and it's much more than a mere physical workout. For the deepest benefits, do it as a devotional offering of your spinal energies to the spiritual eye, the "inner sun": alternately inhale into a backward bend to *lift* energy toward the brain, then exhale into a forward bend to *relax* the spinal energies toward the brain. If you can make those movements of energy your primary focus, all the better. Practice Surya Namaskar slowly, gracefully, and reverently, with the spirit of the affirmation flowing through all your movements:

> *"Salutations to the sun, to the awakening light within,*
> *to the dawning of higher consciousness in all beings."*

Technique

Breathe and move slowly and smoothly throughout this sequence; never hurry. Practice the alignments points given elsewhere for the individual positions. If it's distracting to use the affirmation during the sequence, then practice it before you begin, and retain the *feeling* of the affirmation as you move through the sequence.

Position 1: Begin in Pranamasana (Salutation Pose), standing with your palms together at the heart. Mentally repeat the affirmation one or more times.

Inhale as you sweep your hands overhead, stretching up into Position 2: a gentle backward bend. Tuck your pelvis as needed to avoid overarching the lower back.

Exhale as you release forward into Position 3: Padahastasana (Hand-to-the-Foot Pose).

Inhale as you bend your right knee and step your left foot back; bring your left knee to the floor, toes pointing backward, and your right knee directly above the right ankle. Finish your inhalation by bringing your hands up overhead, palms facing each other in Position 4: Banarasana (Monkey Pose), which is like Virabhadrasana I (Warrior Pose I) except that the left knee is on the floor.

Retain your breath as you bring your hands to the floor, step your right foot back alongside the left, and hold your body briefly in Position 5, the Plank Pose.

Exhale as you lower yourself into Position 6: Ashtanga Namaskar (Eight-Limbed Salutation), in which the feet, knees, hands, chest, and chin are touching the floor.

As you inhale, slide forward and up into Position 7: Bhujangasana (Cobra Pose).

As you exhale, release down and then push back and up into Position 8: Adho Mukha Shvanasana (Downward-Facing Dog Pose).

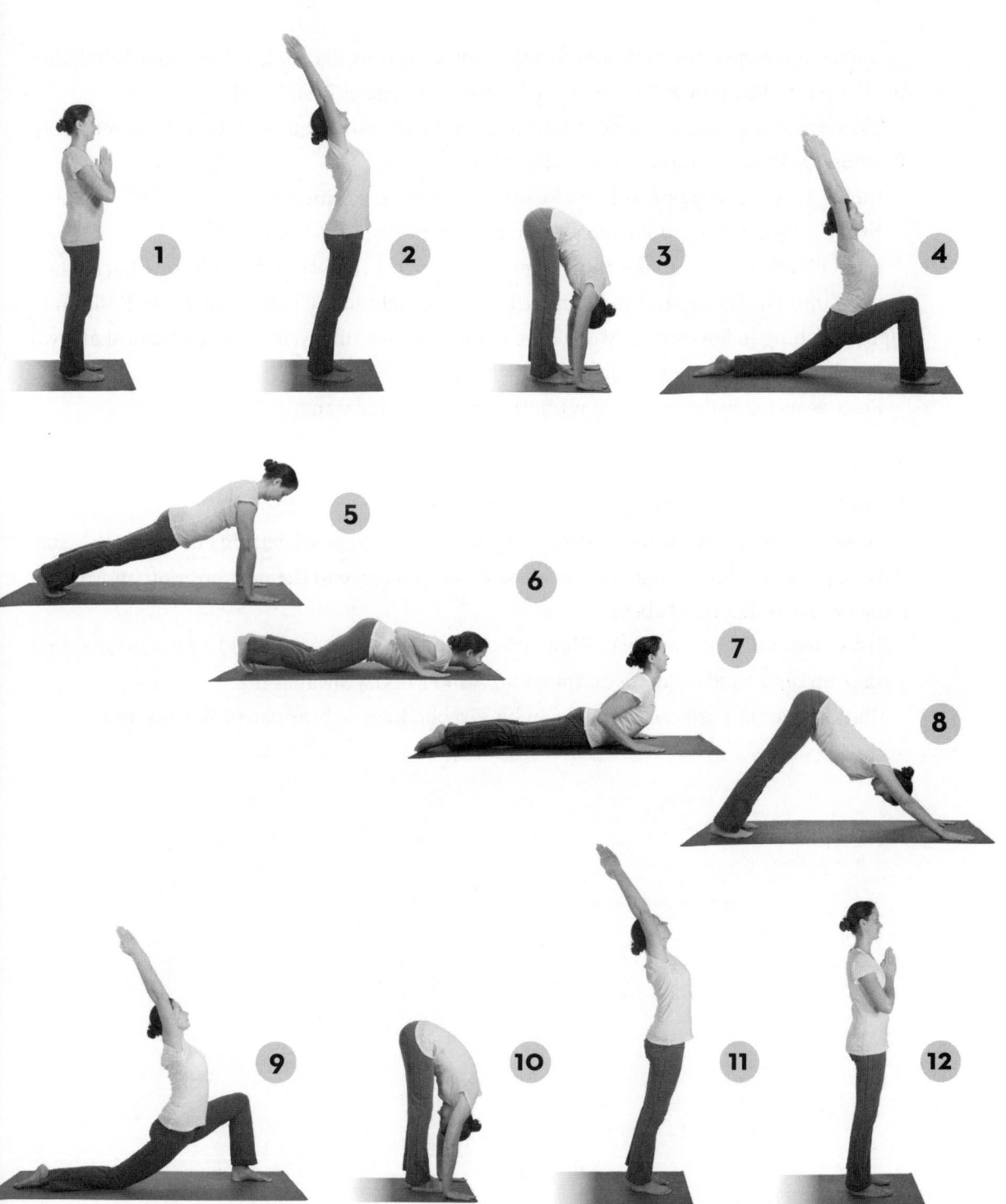

Inhale as you step your left foot forward between your hands, finishing your inhalation by lifting into **Position 9**: Banarasana (the mirror image of Position 4).

Exhale as you bring your hands to the floor and step your right foot forward and relax into **Position 10**: Padahastasana (same as Position 3).

Inhale as you sweep upward into **Position 11** (same as Position 2).

Exhale as you return to **Position 12**: Pranamasana (same as Position 1).

Immediately move through the sequence again; this time step the right foot back when coming into Position 4, and step forward with the right foot when coming into Position 9. Upon finishing in Position 12, you'll have completed one full cycle of Surya Namaskar (two times through the sequence, alternating which foot steps back first).

Practice as many cycles as you wish, then pause in Tadasana.

Variations

Surya Namaskar has many variations. Here are three:

- Easier: For extra stretching and/or strengthening—or to avoid getting out of breath—stay in each position for a number of breaths. When you move to the next position, move with the breath as described above.
- Easier: Instead of moving from Bhujangasana directly into Adho Mukha Shvanasana, first come up onto hands and knees, then into Adho Mukha Shvanasana.
- More advanced: Positions 4 and 9 can be Virabhadrasana I instead of Banarasana.

4.2—FLOOR ASANAS I:
RELEASE ENERGY FROM YOUR EXTREMITIES

By perfect relaxation the whole Yoga science can be mastered. Relaxation must be taken into progressively subtler realms, from physical calmness through mental and emotional calmness to spiritual expansion and receptivity.

—SWAMI KRIYANANDA

Many standing asanas require considerable energy in the shoulders and arms, and of course, all standing asanas require energy in the legs. That, along with the habit-tendency of the arms and legs to want to be "up and doing," can mean that substantial energy may linger in the extremities after the last standing asana. That energy needs to be recalled into the spine.

To do so, in Ananda Yoga we follow the last standing asana with a sequence of floor asanas that stretch your extremities and thereby release the lingering energy. Physical release alone, however, is not enough, because the mind has its own deep-seated tendencies toward physical activity, and those tendencies can continue to send energy to the limbs—without a need for it, without even your awareness of it. Here are some ways to counter those tendencies and be more effective in this stretch-and-release stage of your practice:

Practice Tips

- "Breathe into" the extremities to free up trapped energy and get it moving. Of course, the physical breath can't reach the extremities, but aided by the physical breathing process, your energy and awareness can easily reach and free that energy.
- Visualize the energy releasing from the extremities: see it naturally returning to the astral spine, as though wanting to return home after doing its work.
- Create an "energy magnet" in your astral spine to attract energy there. Simply concentrating there will help. Even better is a brief seated practice of Dirgha Pranayama I (Full Yogic Breath) after your last standing asana: without exaggerating your physical breathing, concentrate on strengthening the astral breath, i.e., the upward and downward flows of energy in the astral spine as you inhale and exhale, respectively.

Janushirasana—Head-to-the-Knee Pose

Life's challenges can cause one to pull back from situations or people—perhaps due to uncertainty, or fear, or reluctance to put out the required energy. Yet solutions come only from giving oneself fully to life, not from pulling back. In Janushirasana, feel the spinal stretch and the wide angle of the thighs opening you not only to a more abundant flow of energy, but also to a greater connection with—and faith in—the goodness of life:

"Left and right and all around—life's harmonies are mine."

Technique

Sit upright with a straight spine and spread your feet wide apart. Bend your right knee, place the sole of the foot against your inner left thigh, and rest your right knee on the floor. Sit evenly on both sitbones. Lengthen forward through your left leg and heel, toes pointing up. If it's difficult to keep your spine straight, sit on the front edge of a cushion and/or bend your left knee slightly. If the right knee doesn't reach the floor, rest it on a cushion.

Active phase: On an inhalation, sweep your hands up the front of your body; stretch tall. Turn to the left leg, and as you exhale, circle your hands out to the sides and down as you fold forward at the hip joints and lengthen out over your left leg, with your spine straight. Rest your hands wherever they reach easily on the floor or left leg, and relax your shoulders. Continue in this position for several breaths: lengthen your spine with each inhalation, and release into a deeper fold at the hip joints (spine still straight) with each exhalation. Walk the hands forward as your torso releases forward.

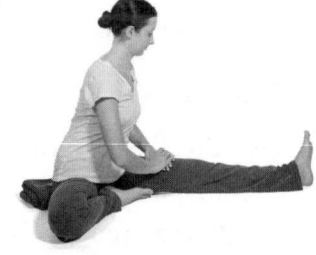

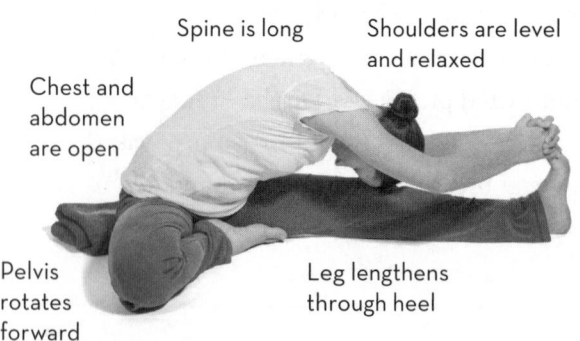

Spine is long   Shoulders are level and relaxed

Chest and abdomen are open

Pelvis rotates forward

Leg lengthens through heel

Relaxation phase: When you've folded forward as far as you can with a straight spine, lengthen your spine with one last inhalation, then exhale and relax into the completed asana. Let your spine round if it's healthy and there's no discomfort. Walk your hands a comfortable distance forward; if they reach your left foot, interlace your fingers and circle them around your left big toe; otherwise, rest your hands on your leg or on the floor. Keep your shoulders level with each other. Go deeper into the forward bend only through relaxation, not through effort.

Breathe smoothly and naturally, mentally affirming, *"Left and right and all around—life's harmonies are mine."*

To exit, walk your hands back in until your spine straightens, then inhale and stretch tall. Exhale into a comfortable sitting position. Pause briefly, then repeat on the other side.

Variations

- Easier: Do the asana with the straight leg directly in front of you rather than off to the side. Because this variation doesn't involve a twist of the spine (as does the standard asana), it's easier to keep the spine straight and the shoulders level.
- Easier: In the active phase of the asana, loop a strap around the ball of your left foot; gently pull on the strap, toward you and slightly down. Engage your spinal muscles so that this gentle pulling will not round your spine, but rather will help you fold forward farther at the hip joints. As you exhale into the relaxation phase, let go of the strap.

Paschimotanasana—Posterior-Stretching Pose

Attitudes of resistance, anxiety, and fear induce physical tensions in the backs of the legs (the urge to run away), tensions that in turn reinforce those attitudes. By stretching away those tensions, Paschimotanasana removes that reinforcement, thereby making it easier to release the underlying attitudes. Set your mind to the task of fully releasing those attitudes, as you affirm,

"I am safe. I am sound. All good things come to me; they give me peace!"

Technique

Sit upright with a straight spine, legs straight in front of you. Lengthen forward through the heels, toes pointing up. If it's difficult to keep your spine straight, sit on the front edge of a cushion and/or bend your knees slightly.

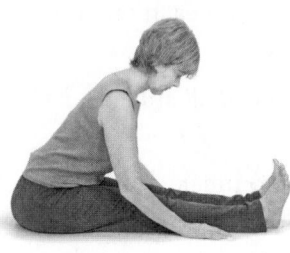

Active phase: On an inhalation, sweep your hands up the front of your body; stretch tall. As you exhale, circle your hands out to the sides and down as you fold forward at the hip joints and lengthen out over your legs, with your spine straight. Rest your hands wherever they reach easily on the floor or legs. Relax your shoulders down away from your ears. Continue in this position for several breaths: lengthen your spine with each inhalation, and release into a deeper fold at the hip joints (spine still straight) with each exhalation. Walk the hands forward as your torso releases forward.

Relaxation phase: When you've folded forward as far as you can with a straight spine, lengthen your spine with one last inhalation, then exhale and relax into the completed asana. Let your spine round if it's healthy and there's no discomfort. Walk your hands a comfortable distance forward; if they reach the feet, wrap the first two fingers of each hand around the corresponding big toe. Go deeper into the forward bend only through relaxation, not through effort.

Spine is long   Head and shoulders relax

Chest and
abdomen
are open

Pelvis
rotates
forward

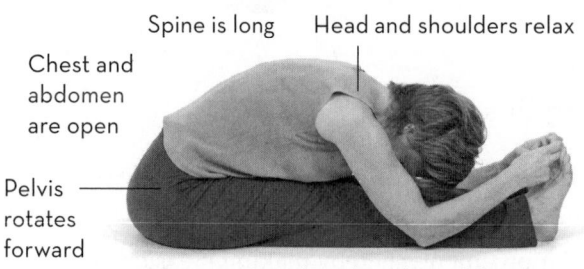

Legs lengthen through heels

Breathe smoothly and naturally, silently affirming, *"I am safe. I am sound. All good things come to me; they give me peace!"*

To exit, walk your hands back in until your spine straightens, then inhale and stretch overhead to lengthen your spine. Exhale into a comfortable sitting position, and pause.

Variation

• Easier: In the active phase of the asana, loop a strap around the balls of your feet; gently pull on the strap, toward you and slightly down. Engage your spinal muscles so that this gentle pulling will not round your spine, but rather will help you fold forward farther at the hip joints. As you exhale into the relaxation phase, let go of the strap.

Baddha Konasana—Bound Angle Pose (aka Butterfly Pose)

On the physical level, Baddha Konasana opens the hips and spine. On a deeper level, this stretch releases energy that's stuck at the base of the astral spine in the first chakra, often due to insecurity, stubbornness, overprotection, mental heaviness, or resentment of—and resistance to—change. Also use your breath, concentration, and visualization to release any such trapped energy as you affirm,

"Secure in my Self, I accept whatever is."

Technique

Sit upright with a straight spine, knees bent and feet flat on the floor. Release your knees out to the sides toward the floor, and bring the soles of the feet together, heels as close to the groin as comfortable. Place cushions under the knees if they don't reach the floor and are uncomfortable.

Interlace the fingers around the toes (or hold your ankles) and pull lightly toward the groin to keep the pelvis level and spine straight. Press the soles of the feet together. If it's difficult to keep the spine straight, sit on the front edge of a cushion.

Active phase: On an exhalation, fold forward at the hips, spine still straight. Continue in this position for several breaths. Lengthen your spine with each inhalation, release into a deeper fold at the hip joints (pelvis tilting forward, spine still straight) with each exhalation.

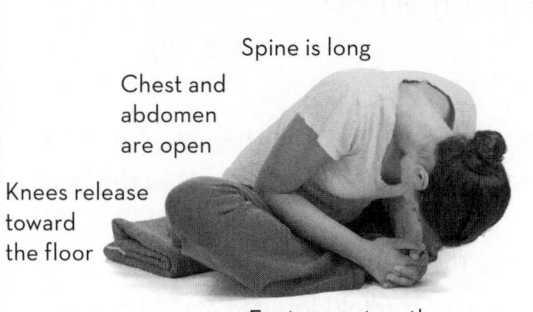

Spine is long

Chest and abdomen are open

Knees release toward the floor

Feet press together

Relaxation phase: When you've folded forward as far as you can with a straight spine, lengthen your spine with one last inhalation, then exhale and relax into the completed asana. Let your spine round if it's healthy and there's no discomfort. Go deeper into the forward bend only through relaxation, not through effort.

Breathe smoothly and naturally, mentally affirming, *"Secure in my Self, I accept whatever is."*

To exit, straighten your spine, then inhale and return to upright. Exhale into a comfortable sitting position, and pause.

Variation

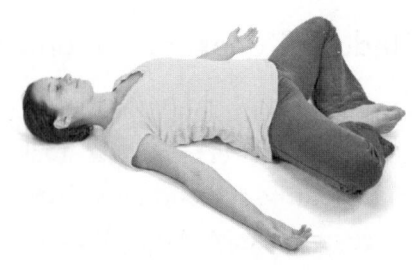

- Supta Baddha Konasana (Supine Bound Angle Pose: different asana, similar energy release, same affirmation): From the upright position before the forward bend, place your hands behind you and slowly lower your back onto the floor, tucking your pelvis as needed to avoid bending your lumbar spine backward too far. Relax your arms out to your sides on the floor, palms facing up. To come out of the asana, use your hands to lift your knees together, and squeeze them into your torso. Straighten your legs and pause in Savasana (Corpse Pose).

Upavistha Konasana—Seated Angle Pose

The open angle of the legs in this asana both reflects and promotes an attitude of conscious acceptance of whatever life brings you—easy or difficult, pleasant or unpleasant. Take acceptance a step farther: keep the chest and heart open, and reach out through the legs, as though actively *welcoming* whatever comes. It is, after all, divinely intended for you. It's not always easy to hold such attitudes, but it's easier when your very posture reinforces them, and easier still when you affirm deeply,

"I welcome every opportunity for further growth."

Technique

Sit upright with a straight spine, and open your legs wide. Lengthen out through your heels, with toes pointing directly upward. If it's difficult to keep your spine straight, sit on the front edge of a cushion.

Active phase: On an inhalation, sweep your hands up the front of your body; stretch tall. As you exhale, circle your hands out to the sides and down as you fold forward at the hip joints

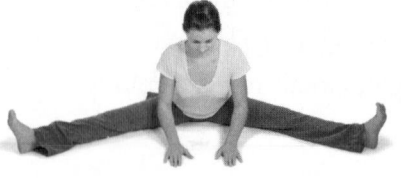

and lengthen out over your legs, with your spine straight. Rest your hands on the floor, wherever they reach easily. Continue in this position for several breaths; lengthen your spine with each inhalation, release into a deeper fold (spine still straight) with each exhalation. Walk the hands forward as your torso releases forward, or if you like, press the fists into the floor beside your hips to help lengthen your spine as you release forward.

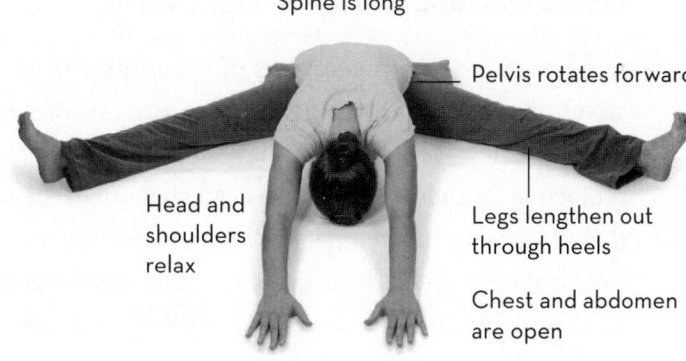

Spine is long

Pelvis rotates forward

Head and shoulders relax

Legs lengthen out through heels

Chest and abdomen are open

Relaxation phase: When you've folded forward as far as you can with a straight spine, lengthen your spine with one last inhalation, then exhale and relax into the completed asana. Let your spine round if it's healthy and there's no discomfort. Walk the hands out as far as comfortable. Go deeper into the forward bend only through relaxation, not through effort.

Breathe smoothly and naturally, silently affirming, "*I welcome every opportunity for further growth.*"

To exit, walk your hands back in and straighten your spine, then inhale and stretch tall. Exhale into a comfortable sitting position, and pause.

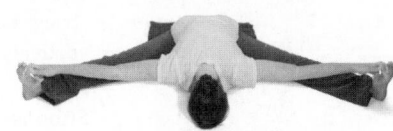

Variation

• More advanced: Bring the chest and/or forehead to the floor, and/or circle the first two fingers of each hand around the corresponding big toe.

Gomukhasana—Face-of-Light Pose[7]

Life presents us with countless opportunities to feel fear, and the more we protect our-selves, the more we confine the heart to an ever-smaller space. Our very posture will reflect this tendency—the shoulders roll in and the chest closes—which in turn reinforces the protective attitude; together they can shut down the heart. Gomukhasana helps you remove that physical reinforcement and thereby begin to free the heart's boundless energy—which in truth, never needs protection. Breathe deeply into the area of the heart, open the chest and shoulders, and add the power of your mind, affirming,

"Free in my heart, I live without fear."

Technique

Sit with your knees bent, your feet flat on the floor in front of you. Slide your left foot under the right knee and place the heel just outside the right hip; bring the left knee to the floor. Lift your right foot and place the heel just outside the left hip. Rest the right knee atop the left. Sit on a cushion if this position stretches your hips uncomfortably.

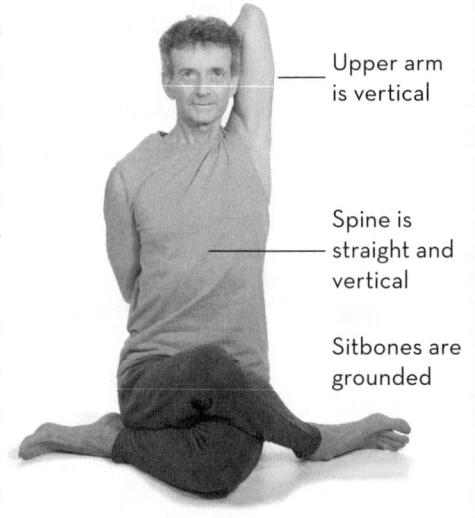

Upper arm is vertical

Spine is straight and vertical

Sitbones are grounded

Bring your right arm behind your back, bend the elbow, and reach the fingers upward along the spine. Stretch your left arm overhead, bend the elbow, and reach the left hand down toward the right hand. Curl the fingers of both hands and interlock them. If the fingers don't reach, join the hands via a strap.

Your left upper arm should be vertical, your head upright. Don't allow your spine to bend to the right; keep it straight, lift the chest, and roll the shoulders open.

Lift your gaze toward the spiritual eye—eyes open or closed—and concentrate in the heart as you breathe smoothly and naturally, mentally affirming, *"Free in my heart, I live without fear."*

To exit, release the arms and interlace your fingers on your right knee, or rest your hands

---

7 You might hear this asana called Cow's-Face Pose, because in modern Sanskrit the word *go* is usually translated as "cow." In ancient Sanskrit, however, *go* means "inner light." Big difference!

on the soles of the feet. Pause in this knee-over-knee sitting position. Then reverse the positions of the legs and repeat on the other side.

Variation

• Easier: On the first side, hold opposite elbows behind your back: left hand holds right elbow, and right hand holds left elbow. On the second side, interchange the positions of the legs and hold opposite elbows overhead.

Sasamgasana—Hare Pose

Sasamgasana entails not only a bodily position, but also a dynamic opposition between a forward-striving spine and a restraining grip on the heels. That opposition helps to magnetize the astral spine, and thereby attract more energy there, which in turn helps you to be more centered, more in control of your energy. Hare Pose also stretches the upper body, brings energy to the brain, and banishes mental fatigue. As you hold the asana, affirm with calm certainty,

"I am master of my energy, I am master of myself."

Technique

From Balasana (Child Pose), grasp your heels, with palms facing each other, thumbs along the outer edges of the feet, and fingers curling onto the insteps.

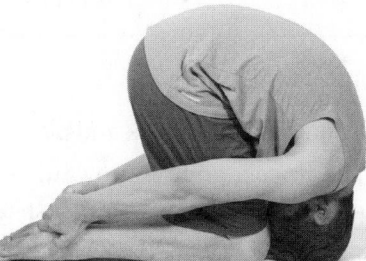

Reach forward through spine

Shoulders, upper arms, and upper back relax

Crown of head rests lightly on floor

Hands firmly grip heels

Bring your forehead toward your knees. On an inhalation, lift your buttocks to bring the crown of your head to the floor and stretch your arms straight. Almost all the weight should remain on your legs; rest only lightly on the crown of your head. Relax your arms, shoulders, and upper back so that they can be stretched and opened. (If you have long arms, position your head farther from your knees for a better stretch.) Use the strength of the legs to power the forward reach of your spine, while your firm grip on the heels prevents actual forward movement.

Breathe smoothly and naturally as this dynamic resistance magnetizes your spine. Mentally affirm, *"I am master of my energy, I am master of myself."*

To exit, exhale as you relax into Balasana.

Variations

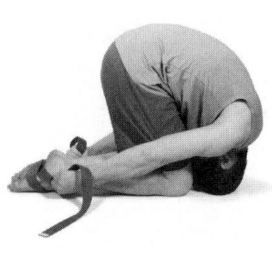

- Easier: If you cannot reach your heels, you can clasp your hands behind your thighs instead. Better still, run a strap under the feet, and bring the ends between the feet and out around the sides. Hold both ends in one hand, and roll to your opposite side, then into Balasana. Separate the ends of the strap into your two hands, and grip the strap as close as possible to the heels, with palms facing toward each other, thumbs toward the floor. Come up into Sasamgasana, with your elbows straight.

Supta Vajrasana—Supine Firm Pose

This asana gives the thighs a deep stretch, helping to squeeze out chronic tensions and restless "get up and go" tendencies that tend to accumulate there. In addition, Supta Vajrasana's backward-bending aspect energizes the spine. Don't let either aspect become an intense experience: use props as needed so that the asana will be pleasant, comfortable, and calming. Relax the mind, too, into freedom from restless activity, as you affirm,

> *"Energetic movement or unmoving peace:*
> *The choice is mine alone! The choice is mine!"*

Technique

From Vajrasana, lean back and place your palms on the floor behind you, shoulder-width apart with the fingers pointing toward your feet. Slowly bend your elbows and lower your torso toward the floor, tucking your pelvis as needed to prevent your lumbar spine from bending backward too far. Your thighs should be parallel and knees on the floor throughout this asana. When you reach your farthest comfortable stretch, soften your neck into the same gentle backward curve as the rest of your spine; don't let the neck bend back sharply.

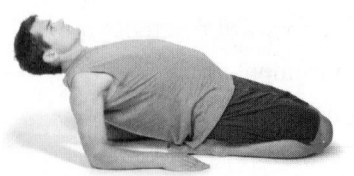

If your elbows easily reach the floor, and if you want to go deeper into the asana, slide your elbows toward your hips and lower your shoulders toward the floor.

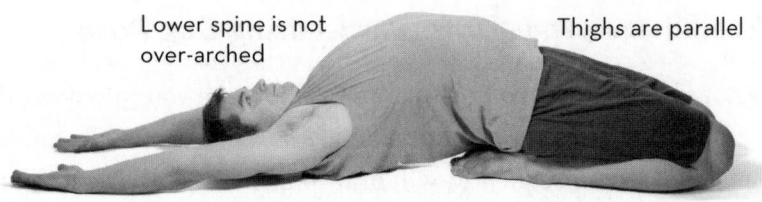

Lower spine is not over-arched

Thighs are parallel

Knees and ankles are not strained

Knees are on floor

If you're able to bring your shoulders to the floor without strain, stretch your arms overhead along the floor, or interlace your fingers behind your head.

However far you descend, your stretch should be comfortable; use props—and restraint—so that you don't strain your ankles, knees, thighs, or spine. Focus on releasing the tops of the thighs, where restless energy tends to accumulate.

Breathe smoothly and naturally, silently affirming, *"Energetic movement or unmoving peace: the choice is mine alone! The choice is mine!"*

To exit, bring your chin toward your chest, roll onto one side, and straighten both legs. Then roll onto your back and hug your knees to your torso. Pause in Savasana (Corpse Pose).

Variations

• Easier: Place cushions under your back and head, and lower yourself onto the cushions. Turn your palms upward by your sides, or bring your arms overhead along the floor—whichever you find more relaxing and peaceful.

• For ankle discomfort: Place a rolled towel under the fronts of your ankles.

• For knee discomfort: Place a cushion between your buttocks and ankles. Don't try to bring your shoulders to the floor, because that would require overarching your lumbar spine.

Adho Mukha Shvanasana—Downward-Facing Dog Pose

Once you learn to be comfortable in this asana, it can take you into deep, dynamic calmness. In addition to stretching the shoulders and legs, Adho Mukha Shvanasana is a partial inversion; subtle gravity, consequently, will draw prana to the brain if you keep your spine straight. Therefore always maintain a straight spine in this asana, even if you need to bend your knees in order to do so. Then the affirmation will come to life:

"Calmness radiates from every fiber of my being."

Technique

Begin on hands and knees: the knees are beneath the hips, and the hands are shoulder-width apart in front of the shoulders, with fingers spread apart and middle fingers pointing forward.

Curl your toes under. On an exhalation, push up and back through your arms and legs, with your spine straight.

Straighten your knees as much as possible without rounding your spine. Keep your neck long and in line with the rest of your spine. Align your arms with your spine, biceps alongside your ears. Broaden across your shoulders and upper back, and roll your shoulders open, away from your ears, so that there's ample space between your upper arms and your head. Press the base of each finger and thumb firmly into the floor. Relax your heels toward the floor; it's fine if they don't reach the floor.

Breathe smoothly and naturally, silently affirming, *"Calmness radiates from every fiber of my being."*

Exit into Balasana (Child Pose) on an exhalation, and pause.

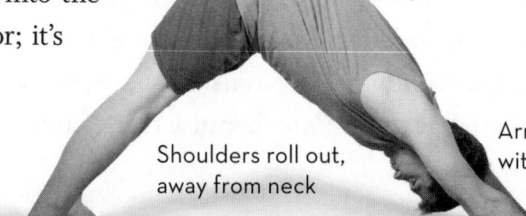

Spine is straight

Shoulders roll out, away from neck

Arms align with spine

Heels release downward   Base of fingers press into floor

Variations

• For wrist discomfort: Place a wedge under the heels of your palms to decrease the angle at which the wrists are bent. Or come onto your fists (palms facing each other) instead of onto the palms. Or bring your forearms to the floor, shoulder-width apart and parallel; this option takes the wrists out of the pose altogether, although it may tax your shoulder flexibility.

4.3—FLOOR ASANAS II: STRETCH AND OPEN YOUR SPINE

The energy-flow in the body can be strengthened by self-effort in two ways: blockages in the nerves can be eliminated, and the flow of energy itself can be increased. Both of these ends may be accomplished by the diligent practice of Hatha Yoga. It is perhaps for this reason above all that Hatha Yoga is termed a science, not merely an art.

—SWAMI KRIYANANDA

Having centered your awareness in the astral spine through the standing asanas, and withdrawn energy from the extremities through the initial floor asanas, you'll next open the astral spine, i.e., stretch it and remove energy blockages so that it can carry more energy to the brain.

To accomplish these aims, you'll stretch the physical spine—and thereby the astral spine as well—in various ways: bend it forward, backward, and sideways, as well as twist it. Although you may already have practiced some of these movements earlier in your routine, they now become the focus. As you practice these asanas, visualize the astral spine becoming an ever-wider, ever-more-open channel, able to carry more energy.

Among other benefits, these movements will help the physical breath to flow more freely and abundantly, which in turn helps prana to flow more freely and abundantly in the astral spine. You can prove these effects to yourself with a simple exercise:

> Sit upright, close your eyes, and notice the degree of ease of your physical breathing. Notice also how freely the astral breath is moving. Next, practice just four of the asanas in this section: a forward bend of the spine, a backward bend, a sideways bend, and finally a twist. Then sit in the initial position once again, close your eyes, and observe your breathing; notice how much easier your breathing has become, and how much more freely the energy flows through the astral spine.

Practice Tips

- Stay as relaxed as possible, even in asanas that require considerable effort. If needed, avoid strain by choosing an easier variation.
- Keep the spine long. Don't bend it to such an extreme that it feels compressed or shortened.
- Never force a stretch. Forcing will diminish your awareness of energy; it also can injure

you. Simply notice where there's resistance to the stretch, then try to exhale away that resistance so that you can *relax* into a deeper stretch.

- Stay aware of the astral breath. Look for small shifts of your bodily position that will help the astral breath to flow more freely.

Parighasana—Gate Pose

Gate Pose enhances your awareness of the spinal energy currents and helps those currents flow more freely, more abundantly. When you view those currents as the core of the experience—use your feeling and visualization faculties—Parighasana becomes a joyous inward dance of prana, a celebration of rising energy. Bring your mind fully into that celebration, affirming,

"Waves of joy surge upward in my spine."

Technique

Kneel on the floor (on a cushion, if needed for knee comfort), with knees hip-width apart, toes pointing behind. Stretch your left leg directly to the left, heel on floor. In order to do this, you may need to rotate your right hip forward a bit. Your chest, however, should face forward. Keep your right thigh vertical and point your left kneecap upward. Bring your left toes to the floor if it's comfortable to do so.

Inhale as you circle your right arm out to the right and overhead. As you exhale, fold sideways at the left hip joint and arc your spine to the left; slide your left hand lightly down the leg to wherever it reaches comfortably. Do not rest much weight on your left hand; use it to stabilize your body, and take care not to hyperextend your left knee. Bring your right arm alongside your right ear, with the right palm facing the left foot. Relax your right shoulder away from your right ear.

Body does not lean forward or back, or twist

Spine is in a long, uniform, sideways arc

No upper body weight rests on hand

Foot presses down

Actively lengthen your spine in its sideways arc; don't bend so far to the left that you inhibit your breathing, because that would also inhibit the energy flow. Face your chest directly forward, and do not lean forward or backward. Ideally, your left leg will be in the same plane as your chest. Keep your neck in the same arc as the rest of your spine. Gaze forward or, if you like, rotate your head to gaze upward past the right upper arm (do not gaze toward the right hand).

Press down through the left foot, and actively lengthen up and to the left through the entire left side of your body, thereby invigorating the left side and opening the right side.

Breathe smoothly and naturally, mentally affirming, "Waves of joy surge upward in my spine."

To exit, inhale and stretch up with the right hand, then return to the initial kneeling position, or relax down into Vajrasana (Firm Pose). Pause, then repeat on the other side.

Ardha Matsyendrasana—Half Spinal Twist

This twist brings prana up the spine into the heart chakra, helping to awaken feelings of love and compassion. Once that prana reaches the heart, however, the bodily position—plus the heart's long-held habit of reaching outside itself for fulfillment—predisposes the energy to move outward rather than to continue upward to the brain. Therefore, use that outward direction in a spiritually useful way: feel it *expanding* your awareness and sympathies, instead of scattering them, and affirm,

"I radiate love and goodwill to soul-friends everywhere."

Technique

Sit with your legs in front of you, knees bent. Slide your right foot under your left knee and place the heel just outside your left hip. Rest your right knee on the floor directly in front of your navel. Cross your left foot over your right knee and place the foot flat on the floor. If the left sitbone rises off the floor, place a cushion under both sitbones to level the pelvis. Place your left hand on the floor behind you, and your right hand on the left knee.

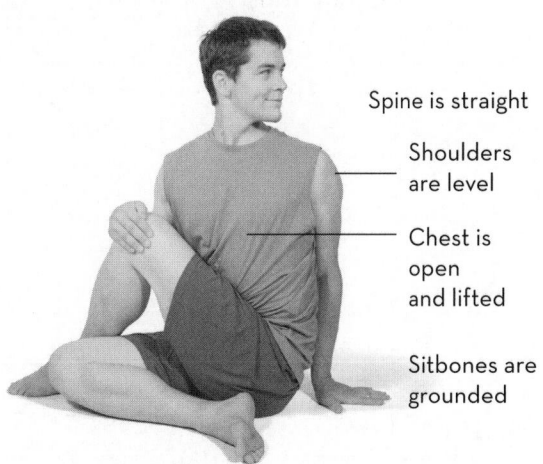

Spine is straight

Shoulders are level

Chest is open and lifted

Sitbones are grounded

Keep your shoulders level and relaxed as you twist: inhale as you press down through your left arm to lengthen your spine, and exhale as you twist to your left in your lower spine. Move the twist progressively up your spine over a number of breaths: lengthen as you inhale, twist as you exhale; finish with your neck, turning your head to gaze past the left shoulder. Use your trunk and spinal muscles to twist; don't force the twist by pulling hard with your right arm. As you twist farther, hook your right elbow around your left knee. If you're able to twist quite far without rounding your spine, bring your right arm to the outside of your left knee, elbow bent and fingers pointing up.

Breathe smoothly and naturally, silently affirming, *"I radiate love and goodwill to soul-friends everywhere."*

To exit, inhale and lengthen the spine, then exhale and slowly untwist. Rest the left knee atop the right, and either interlace your fingers on your left knee, or rest your hands on the soles of the feet. Pause, then reverse the positions of the legs and repeat on the other side.

Variations

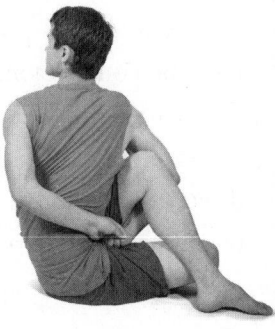

- Easier: If your right hip is tight, you can leave your right leg straight on the floor. If your left hip is tight, slide your left foot farther away from you, or place your left foot against your right shin rather than crossing it over your right knee.
- More advanced: Once you get fully into the twist, wrap your right arm around the outside of your left knee, then under the knee, and join your hands behind you. Keep your chest open and spine straight, and don't force the twist by applying significant leverage with your arms.

Jathara Parivartanasana—Supine Twist

Like all twists, this asana opens the astral spine so that more energy can flow to the brain. You might feel that opening most clearly *after* the asana. While you're *in* the asana, fix your attention on the central axis of every twist: the astral spine. If your breathing feels a bit squeezed by the twist, try to bring a sense of relaxation and spaciousness into the center of the torso; that will both free your breathing and help open the astral spine, as you silently affirm,

"I open to the flow of God's life within me."

Technique

Lie on your back, legs parallel and spine long. Bend your left knee and slide the foot in. Press the foot into the floor to lift your buttocks and shift them to the left; then lower your weight onto the right buttock. Place your left foot on top of your right thigh, just above the knee.

Reach your left arm out to your left, palm facing up. Place your right hand on your left knee. Inhale and lengthen your spine, then as you exhale, slowly roll your lower body to the right on your right hip, keeping your left shoulder blade on the floor. Use your right hand to guide the twist, not to force it.

Move the twist slowly up your spine; actively lengthen through the spine and right leg. When you reach the limit of your twist, lift your head slightly, rotate it to your left, and then place it back on the floor. Your left knee need not reach the floor.

Breathe length and openness into your entire spine, mentally affirming, *"I open to the flow of God's life within me."*

To exit, roll onto your back once again, shift your hips back to center, and straighten your left leg on the floor. Pause in Savasana (Corpse Pose), then repeat on the other side.

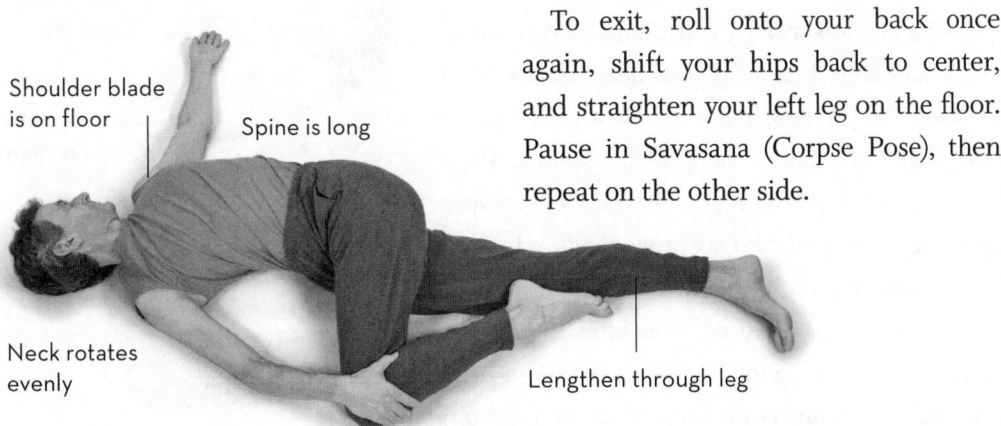

Shoulder blade is on floor

Spine is long

Neck rotates evenly

Lengthen through leg

Variation

• More advanced: Once you have entered the twist, straighten the top (left) leg and either hold the left foot with your right hand, or loop a strap around the ball of the left foot and hold the strap with your right hand. Bring the foot toward the head, keeping the leg straight. This deepens the stretch of the left hip and adds a stretch of the left leg.

Ustrasana—Camel Pose

Relax, yet also lengthen, into a progressively deeper backward bend. Lift through the front of the torso throughout Ustrasana; sagging backward is unsafe for your spine as well as less beneficial on the levels of energy and consciousness. Lift and open especially in the heart region—as a flower lifts and opens to the sun—affirming,

"With calm faith, I open to Thy light."

Technique

Kneel on the floor (on a cushion, if needed for knee comfort), with knees and feet hip-width apart, toes pointing behind. Place the heels of your palms on the back rim of the pelvis, fingers pointing down and elbows shoulder-width apart behind you.

Keep your lower body stationary as you inhale into a backward bend; lift your heart up and back to guide the process. Then exhale and relax into that position without sagging backward. Press forward and down with your hands to keep your upper legs vertical and to prevent your lumbar spine from bending backward too far.

On succeeding breaths, continue lifting "up and over the top" into the backward bend until you can place your hands on your heels. Use your

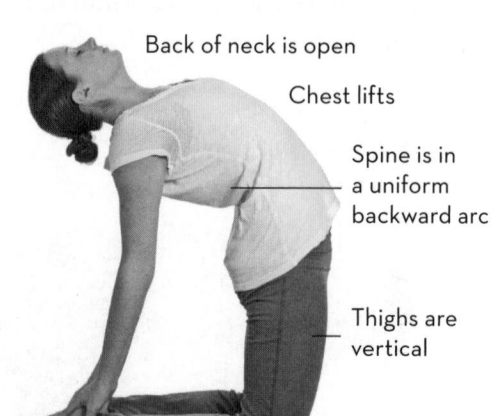

Back of neck is open

Chest lifts

Spine is in a uniform backward arc

Thighs are vertical

inhalations to create length, support, and openness throughout the body, especially in the spine. Use your exhalations to relax—with stability, and without sagging—into your current position.

Continue to lift as you hold the pose; rest only minimal weight on your hands. Keep your neck in the same backward curve as the rest of your spine; don't let your head hang back. If your neck tires, bring your chin toward your chest. Stay as open as possible in the back of your chest, even though your shoulder blades will be squeezed together a bit.

Breathe smoothly and naturally, mentally affirming, "With calm faith, I open to Thy light."

To exit, bring your chin toward your chest, then inhale as you stretch one hand forward and up to pull yourself upright; exhale as you sit back on your heels.

Pause in Vajrasana (Firm Pose) or Balasana (Child Pose).

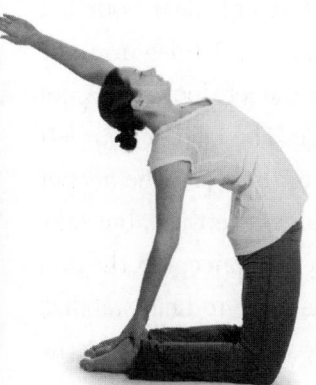

Variations

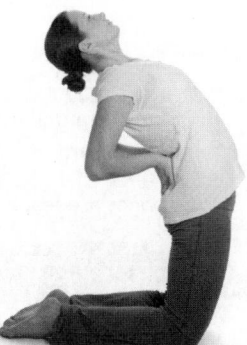

- Ardha Ustrasana (Half Camel Pose): As above, bring your right hand to the right heel but reach up and back with the left arm. Face your torso as forward as possible; try not to twist. After you exit, pause in Vajrasana or Balasana, then repeat on the other side.
- Easier: Keep the heels of your palms on the back rim of the pelvis throughout the asana, pressing forward and down with your hands.

Rajakapotasana—Royal Pigeon Pose

As your spine lifts out of the horizontal plane of your legs—one reaching forward, the other backward—lift your consciousness high above all distractions of the vanished past and the uncertain future. Rise into the only time that's real: right now. Savor the sense of being dynamically awake in—and opening your heart completely to—the fullness of this moment, as you affirm,

"I rise above all thought of past and future, into the Eternal Now."

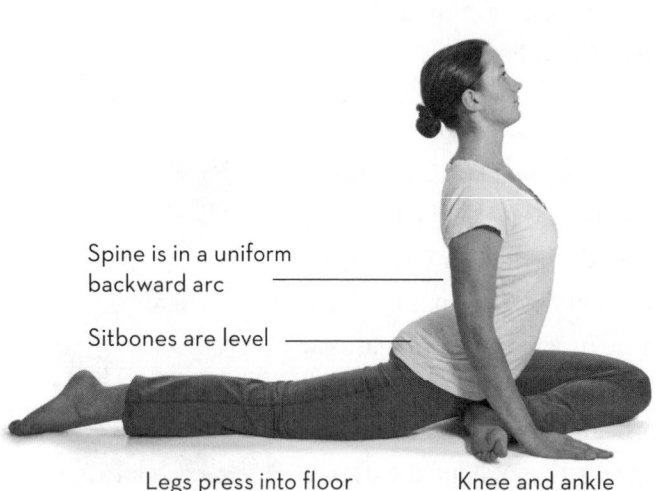

Spine is in a uniform backward arc

Sitbones are level

Legs press into floor

Knee and ankle are not strained

Technique

From a hands-and-knees position, slide your left knee forward, near your left thumb, and rotate your left leg from the hip joint so that the left foot comes out to your right side. The farther your left foot comes out to the right, the deeper is the stretch in your left hip, but take care not to twist your knee; flex the toes back toward the knee to help stabilize it. To relieve any strain or stretch in the left knee (due to a tight left hip), place a cushion under the left thigh.

Slide your right leg back, straightening the knee and bringing the top of the thigh to the floor, toes pointing backward. If your pelvis tips to the left enough to cause discomfort in your spine, place a cushion under the left thigh.

Walk your hands toward you, press your hands and both legs into the floor, and lift through your heart, lengthening your entire spine up into a backward bend. Lift your chin and your gaze without bending your neck back sharply. Relax your shoulders down away from your ears. Tuck your pelvis as needed to prevent your lumbar spine from bending backward too far.

Breathe smoothly and naturally, mentally affirming, *"I rise above all thought of past and future, into the Eternal Now."*

Exit to Balasana (Child Pose) or to a comfortable sitting position. Pause, then repeat on the other side.

Variation

• More advanced: After entering the above position, bend your right knee and interlace the fingers of both hands around the right ankle. Press the right foot back away from you to open your chest and deepen your backward bend, without forcing it, as you continue to lift. Draw your navel toward your spine as needed to prevent your lumbar spine from bending backward too far.

Bhujangasana—Cobra Pose

All backward bends energize the spine, but this basic version of Cobra Pose also lifts the spinal energies toward the brain and vitalizes the will. The key lies both in working with the energy reality of the asana—not just with the muscles—and in practicing the asana with an attitude of calm enthusiasm. Feel yourself ready, willing, and eager to rise to any challenge that may come your way, and affirm,

"I rise joyfully to meet each new opportunity."

Technique

Lie prone with your legs parallel, arms at your sides, and head turned to one side. Lengthen your spine by walking your feet and hips farther away from your head. Then bring your forehead to the floor and place your palms on the floor beside your chest, elbows close to your sides.

You'll rise *slowly* into the asana in three stages, over the course of several breaths. First, as you inhale, lift your head and feel the life-force activating the neck and upper back muscles that do the lifting. Next, feel energy activating the upper and middle back muscles to lift your chest. Finally, press your pubis into the floor, and use your lower back to lift your torso, again with attention to the prana that activates those muscles.

Use your back muscles, not your arms, to rise as high as possible. Keep your elbows close to your sides, shoulders down away from

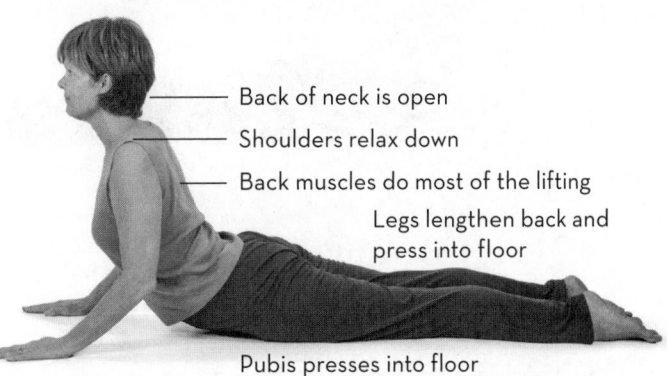

Back of neck is open

Shoulders relax down

Back muscles do most of the lifting

Legs lengthen back and press into floor

Pubis presses into floor

your ears, and shoulder blades spread apart. Lengthen back through the legs, and press legs and feet into the floor to give additional lift. Feel the vibrant energy throughout your spine, with muscles engaged all along its length.

Now, if you like, use your arms to rise farther. Keep your back muscles engaged, and don't bend your spine beyond what's safe and comfortable for you; tuck your pelvis as needed to prevent your lumbar spine from bending backward too far. Gaze softly upward, with your neck in the same graceful backward arc as the rest of your spine.

Breathe smoothly and naturally, silently affirming, *"I rise joyfully to meet each new opportunity."*

As you slowly exit on an exhalation, notice energy releasing first from the lower back, then the middle back, then the upper back, and finally the neck. Feel all that released energy surging toward the brain and bathing it in strength and vitality. Pause in the prone position (head now turned to the other side), or in Balasana (Child Pose), or in Savasana (Corpse Pose).

Variation

• Easier (Sphinx Pose): Place your palms on the floor beside your eyes, with elbows on the floor, close to your sides. Use your back muscles to lift up onto your forearms, so that your upper arms are vertical. Even though you could stay propped up on your arms without using your back muscles at all, strongly engage the back muscles to help energize your spine. This makes the asana more dynamic; it also strengthens the back muscles so that standard Bhujangasana will be easier for you.

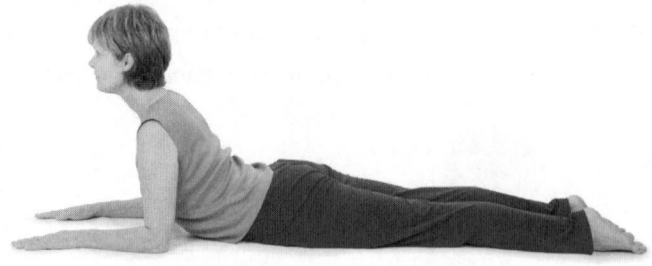

Setu Bandhasana—Bridge Pose

This backward-bending partial inversion both expresses and promotes active self-offering, the primary attitude that draws divine grace. Rather than *pushing* yourself up into the asana, *offer* yourself upward. Invite higher awareness into your heart, into your mind, and into your life, as you affirm,

"I offer every thought as a bridge to divine grace."

Technique

Lie on your back with your knees bent and feet flat on the floor near your buttocks; knees and feet should be hip-width apart. (Experiment to find the foot placement that results in your shins being vertical in the completed asana.) You might wish to lie on a folded blanket in order to cushion your upper vertebrae; if you come up high in this asana, you might need to lie on one or more blankets to avoid overstretch-

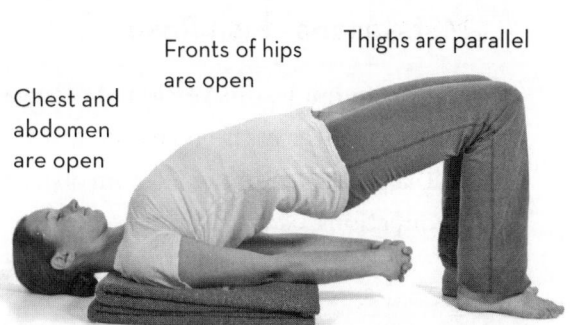

Chest and abdomen are open

Fronts of hips are open

Thighs are parallel

Backs of arms, shoulders, and head press down

ing your neck. See "Practice Tips" in Section 4.5 for details on using a blanket in this way.

On an inhalation, slowly peel your spine off the floor, one vertebra at a time, by pressing down with your feet and the backs of your arms, and by expanding the front of your torso upward. Throughout this asana, keep your thighs and feet parallel (or nearly so), and tuck your pelvis as needed to prevent your lumbar spine from bending backward too far.

Interlace your fingers behind you and roll your shoulders under, one at a time, opening your chest without closing off the back of your torso. Come up as far as comfortable by pressing down with your feet and the backs of your arms and shoulders, and continuing to expand upward with the front of your torso. Also press the back of your head into the floor to open the throat area, which is the bridge between heart and head; don't turn your head.

Breathe smoothly and naturally, silently affirming, *"I offer every thought as a bridge to divine grace."*

To exit, exhale as you slowly lower your spine to the floor, one vertebra at a time. Squeeze your knees briefly into your torso, then pause in Savasana (Corpse Pose).

Variation

• More advanced: You can open a bit more if, once you
have come up and rolled your shoulders under, you separate the hands and grasp your ankles. To avoid straining your knees, practice this variation only if you're
able to keep the lower legs vertical (or nearly vertical).

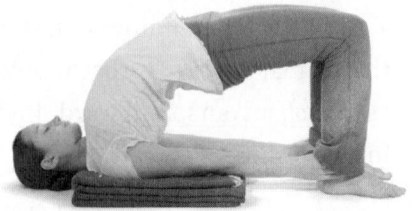

Matsyasana—Fish Pose

Easy though it is, this version of Matsyasana can promote a great deal of opening. The key
is to engage the entire body, not just the upper body. Then the front of the torso and neck
will easily and naturally blossom open. Feel your awareness, too, opening and expanding in
all directions, as you affirm,

"My soul floats on waves of cosmic light."

Technique

Lie on your back with your legs parallel. Place your hands, palms down, underneath your
sitbones, with your arms straight and elbows close to your sides. (If your hands reach past
your sitbones when the arms are straight, then begin with your elbows bent and away from
the body; walk the elbows back in to shoulder-width as you come up into the asana.)

On an inhalation, press your elbows into the floor and your sitbones into your hands;
lift up from your heart, arching your upper body into a backward bend. Lightly rest only
the back corner of your head (not the crown) on the floor, so that your neck doesn't bend
backward sharply.

Maintain a dynamic backward bend—and thereby a dynamic opening of the abdomen,

Front of torso expands

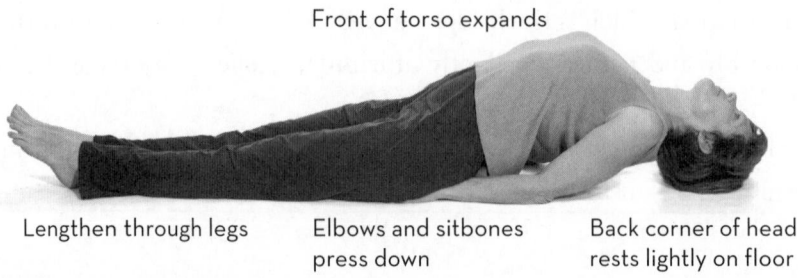

Lengthen through legs   Elbows and sitbones   Back corner of head
                            press down   rests lightly on floor

chest, and neck—by continuing to lengthen the legs, to press the sitbones into the hands and the elbows into the floor, and to lift through the heart.

Breathe smoothly and naturally, feeling both your body and your awareness opening up and expanding, as you silently affirm, *"My soul floats on waves of cosmic light."*

To exit, lift the chin and slowly lower the upper body to the floor, with control. Pause in Savasana (Corpse Pose).

Variation

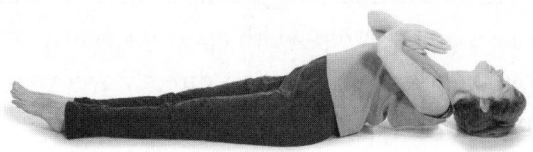

• More advanced (do this only if you have a strong, healthy neck and are *extra* careful not to overarch or overstress the neck): With your legs either straight (as above) or crossed (ideally, in Padmasana, Lotus Pose, but any cross-legged position is okay), remove the supports of your elbows, and rest your weight on the buttocks, the legs, and the back corner of the head. Press down with your legs and with the back of the head. Join the palms at the heart and lift your heart to press against your hands. If you're doing the cross-legged version, you can instead grasp the right toes with the left hand, and the left toes with the right hand.

Chakrasana—Wheel Pose (aka Circle Pose)

It takes energy to do this vitalizing asana, but it can give you even more energy than you put into it. To awaken the most energy, and to avoid straining your joints, try to distribute the backward bend *evenly* throughout the spine, hips, and shoulders. Then you'll feel the body position, breath, energy, and mind together creating a circle of ever-increasing vitality—a circle that will energize you in the asana and sustain you afterward—as you affirm,

"I am awake! Energetic! Enthusiastic!"

Technique

Lie on your back, knees bent and feet on the floor near your buttocks; knees and feet should be hip-width apart. Place your palms on the floor underneath or alongside your shoulders, elbows high and fingers pointing toward your feet and spread apart.

Press down with your feet to slowly lift your pelvis, thighs staying parallel.

Bring your elbows as close as possible to shoulder-width apart; keep them that way as you enter the asana, because that will help stabilize your shoulders and distribute weight evenly on the wrists. On an exhalation, press your hands and feet into the floor, and straighten your arms to lift your upper body. Lead the upward movement with your abdomen, and don't let your elbows or knees splay out to the sides. As you come up, tuck your pelvis as needed to prevent your lumbar spine from bending backward too far.

Relax the fronts of your hips, and walk your feet as close to your hands as possible, with knees and feet hip-width apart (or nearly so). Ideally, your shoulders will end up directly over your hands, and knees directly over your feet. Keep your abdomen high, and relax your neck without bending it back sharply.

As you hold the asana, be especially aware of your spinal energy and overall vitality, not just muscular effort. Breathe smoothly and naturally, silently affirming, *"I am awake! Energetic! Enthusiastic!"*

To exit, exhale as you slowly—with control—bend your elbows and lower your shoulders to the floor, not allowing the elbows to splay out to the sides. Then relax your buttocks to the floor, and squeeze your knees against your torso to release any tension in the lower back. Pause in Savasana (Corpse Pose).

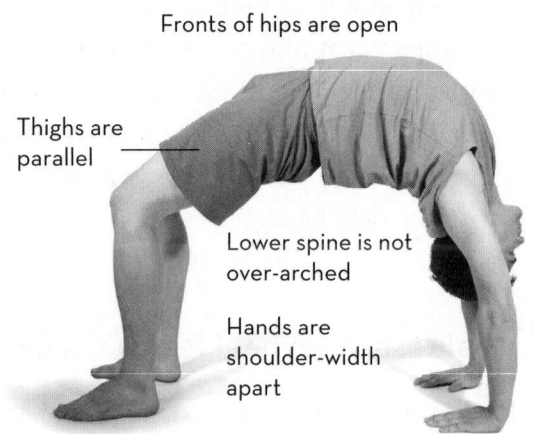

Fronts of hips are open

Thighs are parallel

Lower spine is not over-arched

Hands are shoulder-width apart

Variation

• Easier: If you don't yet have sufficient shoulder strength for the full pose, place your hands on something higher than your feet, e.g., a block or the first or second step of a stairway. For safety, ensure that your block will not slide.

Pavanamuktasana—Wind-Freeing Pose

Although Pavanamuktasana relaxes the legs and physical spine, its main purpose is to help free the energies in the lower astral spine so that they can rise more easily toward the brain. Wrap your arms firmly around your knees to deepen this process of release as you affirm,

"I release my spinal energies to rise in light."

Technique

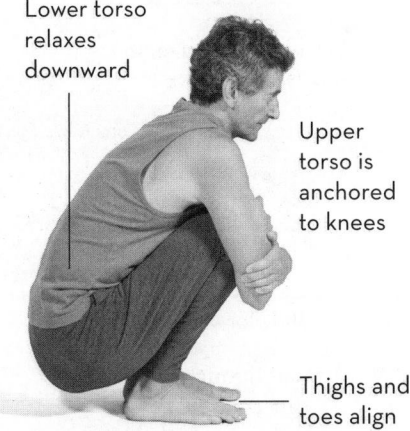

Lower torso relaxes downward

Upper torso is anchored to knees

Thighs and toes align

Squat down fully, with thighs together and heels flat on the floor. Wrap your arms around your knees and hold your chest firmly against your knees to anchor your upper spine in place. Your abdomen, although it will be against your thighs, should feel as free from the legs as possible so that your lower spine can release toward the floor. Maintain length in the back of your neck as you gaze forward.

Your only effort should be in your arms as they anchor the upper spine. Breathe smoothly and naturally, relaxing everything else—especially the legs, torso, buttocks, and pelvic floor. With each exhalation, let your lower physical spine release and lengthen even more, thus freeing more energy in the astral spine. Silently affirm, *"I release my spinal energies to rise in light."*

To exit, sit back on your buttocks and pause in a comfortable sitting position.

Variations

- If comfort requires that your knees be wider apart, then turn your feet out accordingly. You may need to wrap each arm individually around—or atop—a knee in order to anchor your upper spine so that the lower spine can release as described above.
- Easier: If it's a struggle to remain upright with heels flat on the floor, place a folded blanket under your heels. Be sure that your buttocks don't touch the blanket, as doing so would inhibit the spinal release.
- For knee discomfort: Lie on your back, bend your knees, and lift your legs toward the chest. Wrap your arms *behind* your knees and draw the knees—horizontally—toward your face. Keep the sacrum on the floor so that the lower spine stays relatively straight.

Bakasana—Crane Pose

This expression of Bakasana offers a unique, gravity-aided stretch of the lower spine, which in turn releases energy from the lower astral spine. Since Bakasana is also a partial inversion, the force of subtle gravity will then help to draw that released energy toward the brain. Open your mind to receive the calm power within that energy, and affirm,

"The silent power of the Infinite expands within me."

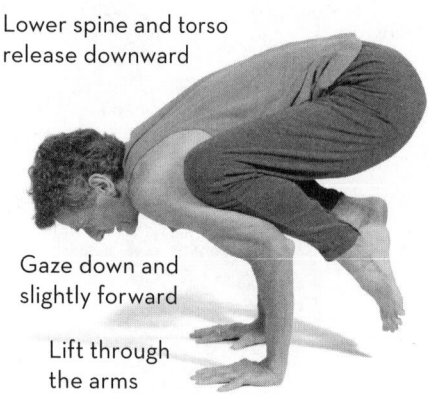

Lower spine and torso release downward

Gaze down and slightly forward

Lift through the arms

Hands shoulder-width apart

Technique

Squat with your feet close to each other, and your knees wide apart. Lean forward with arms between thighs and palms on the floor, shoulder-width apart and middle fingers pointing forward. Bend your elbows and bring your upper arms under your shins.

Rise onto the balls of your feet and slowly lean forward, shifting weight onto the backs of the upper arms until your feet leave the floor and you're balanced, with your shins resting on the backs of your upper arms.

Straighten your arms a bit and keep lifting through the arms rather than allowing weight to settle onto the arms. Look down and slightly forward.

Find your perfect compromise between more stability (which comes from lightly squeezing your inner thighs against your torso) and greater spinal release (which comes from keeping legs relaxed so that their weight will help to stretch open the lower spine).

Breathe smoothly and naturally, mentally affirming, *"The silent power of the Infinite expands within me."*

To exit, slowly lower your feet to the floor, back into the initial squatting position. Then pause in a comfortable sitting position.

Variation

• Easier: Do the asana with your head just above a stable stack of cushions so that you'll both feel more secure and be safer should you lose your balance. It's best to learn the asana with your head resting on some cushions, as shown here.

4.4—FLOOR ASANAS III: ENERGIZE YOUR SPINE

In the practice of the yoga postures, try entertaining the awareness that all the energy of the universe is yours already to command. Open yourself mentally to its inflow, and direct it through your body by the direct exercise of your will. Radiate it also outward, in harmony and blessing to all.

—SWAMI KRIYANANDA

Having opened the astral spine so that it can receive more energy and carry energy more freely to the brain, we now turn to asanas that fill the astral spine with energy and/or lift energy higher in the spine. View these asanas as final preparation for the inverted asanas, which will help draw that spinal energy more completely to the brain.

Practice Tips

- Stay connected with energy; don't let physical effort command *all* your attention. The asana instructions offer tips on how to do this.
- Keep the breath flowing smoothly. That's not easy in some of these asanas, but it's important; it will come with practice. Then you'll be calmer in the midst of physical effort, and it will be easier to focus on energy rather than on effort.
- As always, use easier asana variations when needed. Straining will limit the amount of energy you can draw into the spine as well as your awareness of that energy.

Navasana—Boat Pose

In Navasana, as in other vigorous asanas, the more you focus on energy rather than on physical effort, the more energy you'll receive, and the deeper and more powerful your experience will be. Be aware especially of the currents of energy moving up and down the spine with your inhalations and exhalations; those currents vitalize the entire body. Keep the front of your torso open and lifting as you affirm,

"Within my every breath is infinite power."

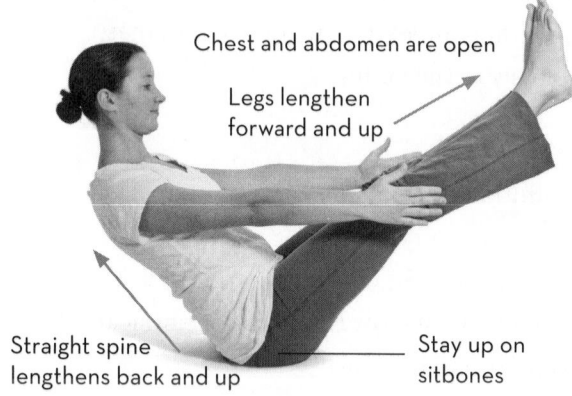

Chest and abdomen are open

Legs lengthen forward and up

Straight spine lengthens back and up

Stay up on sitbones

Technique

Sit upright with knees bent in front of you, feet on the floor. Curl your fingers underneath your knees.

Inhale and lengthen your spine; then as you exhale, straighten your knees (with your hands supporting your legs) and lean back with a straight spine. Your body will form a "V" shape. You may need to bring the chin toward the chest in order to balance. Keep your belly and chest open, and stay up on the backs of your sitbones; don't allow your lower spine to round.

When you've found your balance, remove the support of your hands, and turn the palms toward the knees. Breathe smoothly and naturally, concentrating on the spinal currents as you silently affirm, *"Within my every breath is infinite power."*

Exit to a comfortable sitting position.

Variations

• Easier: Bend your knees slightly and/or continue to support your legs with your hands.
• Easier (Ardha Navasana, Half Boat Pose): Lift just one leg at a time, with the other foot on the floor, knee bent. If you need to, support the raised leg with one or both hands. Pause between sides in a comfortable sitting position.

Akarshana Dhanurasana—Pulling-the-Bow Pose

This pose is powerfully vitalizing—physically (for the lower portion of the torso), energetically (for the spine), and spiritually (for the will). To reap those benefits, keep your spine as straight as possible, your chest open, and your awareness strongly at the point between the eyebrows, as you affirm,

"With shafts of will I pierce the heart of worries."

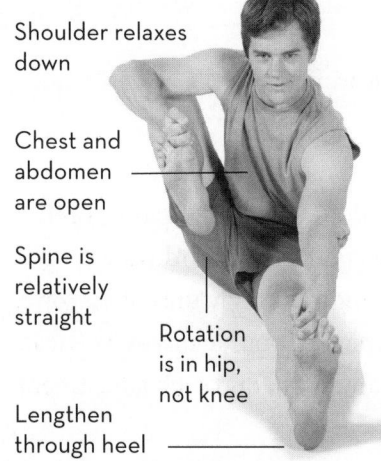

Shoulder relaxes down

Chest and abdomen are open

Spine is relatively straight

Rotation is in hip, not knee

Lengthen through heel

Technique

Sit upright, with the left leg straight in front of you, and right knee bent, right foot on the floor. (Most people need to sit on the front edge of a cushion in order to keep the spine straight in this asana.) Circle the first two fingers of your right hand around the right big toe, or instead hold the entire right foot if that's more comfortable.

Fold forward from your hips, just enough to circle the first two fingers of your left hand around the left big toe. On an inhalation, lift the right foot and pull it back toward the right ear, as though drawing a bow. Keep the right knee close to your torso, your spine as straight as possible, and your right shoulder down away from the right ear, so that the shoulders are more or less level.

Gaze intently ahead, as though aiming an arrow. Or close your eyes and gaze intently at the spiritual eye. Breathe smoothly and naturally, mentally affirming, *"With shafts of will I pierce the heart of worries."*

Exit with control, and pause in a comfortable sitting position. Then repeat on the other side.

Variations

• Easier: To avoid rounding your spine as you bend forward, you can loop a strap around the farther foot and hold the strap instead of the toe.

• More advanced (crossover variation): Grasp the left big toe with the right hand, and the right big toe (or entire right foot) with the left hand. Rotating from the right hip, let the right knee come out to your right and draw the

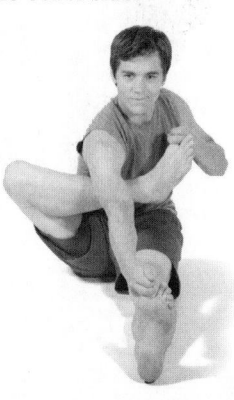

right foot toward your left ear. To avoid twisting the right knee, keep the toes flexed back toward the knee and focus the joint movement of the right leg in the hip joint.

Purvotanasana—Front-Stretching Pose

Rather than *pushing* yourself up into this energizing asana, cultivate the feeling of *expanding* upward with the pelvis, abdomen, and chest—with an attitude of giving yourself wholeheartedly to life, holding nothing back. Use the joyful enthusiasm of the affirmation to help you easily rise up and hold both the position and the attitude:

"With a burst of energy, I rise to greet the world."

Technique

Sit with your legs in front of you, knees bent and feet on the floor. Place your palms on the floor behind your hips, shoulder-width apart, with the fingers pointing toward your feet.

As you inhale, press your hands and feet into the floor, lifting your body until your torso and thighs are horizontal. Walk your feet forward or backward until your arms are vertical. (Experiment to find where to place your hands and feet initially so that no such adjustment is needed.)

Straighten your legs without lowering your torso, and if possible, place your feet flat on the floor. Expand your torso upward into a backward bend as far as possible. Although the physical strength to rise will come from your arms, legs, and back muscles, try to feel that rising comes primarily as a result of expanding upward through the front of your torso.

Relax your head back in line with the gentle backward arc of the rest of the spine; don't drop your head back. (If your neck muscles tire, bring your chin to your chest.)

Breathe smoothly and naturally, silently affirming, *"With a burst of energy, I rise to greet the world!"*

Exit on an exhalation, and pause in a comfortable sitting position.

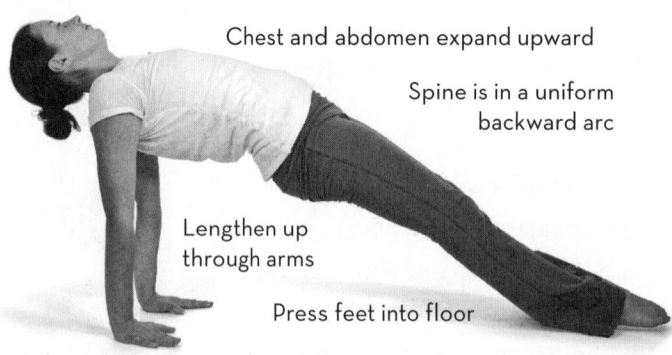

Chest and abdomen expand upward

Spine is in a uniform backward arc

Lengthen up through arms

Press feet into floor

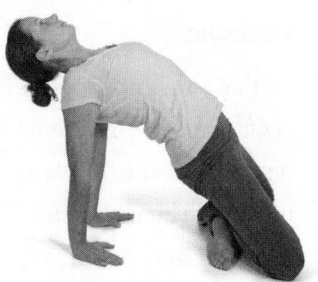

Variation

• Easier: Begin in Vajrasana (Firm Pose) or a cross-legged sitting position, hands on the floor behind you as described above. Lift the pelvis, press the knees into the floor, and expand up into a backward bend. The pelvis and belly will not lift as high as in the standard pose, but the chest should do so.

Salabhasana—Locust Pose

This energizing asana yields the greatest benefits—and becomes easiest—when you enter the pose with the attitude of soaring upward joyfully, as though you were a bird. Then, as you hold the position, feel yourself rising ever higher and more easily with each inhalation, and absorb your mind ever deeper in the affirmation:

"I soar upward on wings of joy!"

Technique

Lie prone with your legs parallel, arms at your sides, and head turned to one side. Lengthen your spine by walking your feet and hips farther away from your head.

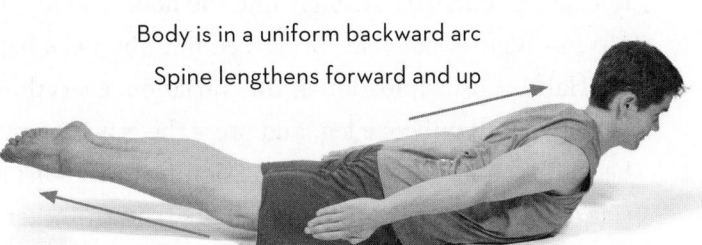

Body is in a uniform backward arc
Spine lengthens forward and up
Legs lengthen back and up   Fingers reach toward feet

Bring your forehead to the floor. Inhale as you press the pubis into the floor and lift the rest of your body—legs, arms, chest, head—off the floor, coming into a backward bend. Turn your palms toward your body or upward, and stretch your fingers toward your feet. Feel that you're not just holding up your body through muscle strength, but rather that you're *lengthening* up into the asana: forward and up through your spine and the crown of your head, and backward and up through your legs. Keep the back of your neck open so that it's in the same gentle backward curve as the rest of your spine.

Breathe smoothly and naturally, mentally affirming, *"I soar upward on wings of joy!"*

Exit on an exhalation, and pause in the prone position (head now turned to the other side), in Balasana (Child Pose), or in Savasana (Corpse Pose).

Variations

- Ardha Salabhasana (Half Locust Pose): Extend your left arm overhead along the floor, right arm down at your side. Lift both arms and the right leg, along with the chest and head. Lead this upward movement with the left arm; don't let the arm lag behind your lifting of the chest and head. After the asana, pause in a prone position, then repeat with the right arm overhead, left arm at your side, and left leg lifting.
- Easier: Same as the preceding variation, but bring the right arm overhead along the floor, and press the right arm and left leg into the floor to help lift the body.
- More advanced: Extend your arms to the sides, as a bird extends its wings, palms down. Or extend your arms directly in front of you, palms facing each other. In either variation, lead the upward movement with your arms; don't let them lag behind your lifting of the chest, head, and legs.
- More advanced (Full Locust Pose): Place your hands on the floor under your hips, with the palms down (or in fists, with the backs of your fists down; or interlace your fingers with thumbs down). The arms are straight. On an inhalation, press your arms strongly into the floor, and lift your legs and lower torso as high as possible. Avoid bending the neck back sharply. (In the Half Locust expression of this variation, everything is the same except you lift only one leg, and press the other leg into the floor to help lift. Try not to twist the spine significantly: don't let one side of the pelvis lift significantly more than the other. After pausing in the prone position, repeat on the other side.)

Dhanurasana—Bow Pose

Dhanurasana gives you a powerful spinal recharge. Although the legs and arms do much to vitalize the body in Bow Pose, also keep your spinal muscles engaged in order to charge your spine with even more energy, and to increase your awareness of that energy. To enhance the effect, affirm,

"I recall my scattered forces to recharge my spine."

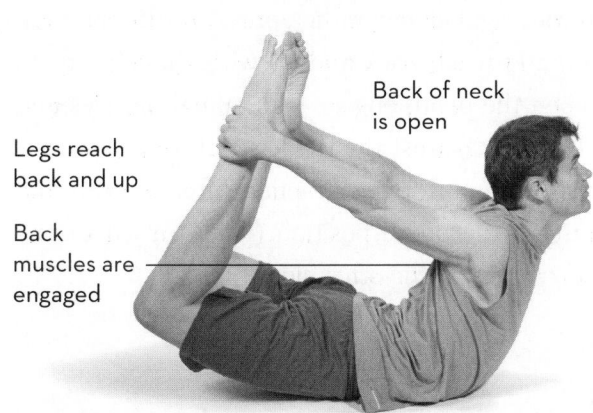

Back of neck is open

Legs reach back and up

Back muscles are engaged

Thighs are parallel

Pubis presses into floor

Technique

Lie prone, legs parallel, arms at your sides and head turned to one side. Lengthen your spine by walking your feet and hips farther away from your head.

Bring your forehead to the floor. Keeping the knees hip-width apart, bend your knees and grasp the outsides of your ankles. To avoid overarching your lower back, press the pubis into the floor throughout this asana.

As you inhale, lift your legs and reach your feet back and up, in order to pull your entire body into a bow shape. To deepen the bend, engage your spinal muscles and pull lightly against the legs with your arms. Keep your shoulder blades spread wide and knees hip-width apart (or nearly so). Gaze upward, with your neck in the same backward curve as the rest of your spine.

Breathe smoothly and naturally, concentrating on the energy pouring into your spine. Silently affirm, *"I recall my scattered forces to recharge my spine."*

Exit to the prone position (head now turned to the other side) or to Balasana (Child Pose), and pause.

Variations

• Easier: If you cannot reach your ankles, loop a strap around your ankles before you lie down: Start with the strap behind your ankles, and wrap the ends of the strap around in front of the ankles, then back between your ankles. Hold both ends in one hand, and roll to your opposite side, then onto your belly. Separate the ends of the strap into your two hands, and grip the strap as close as possible to the ankles, palms facing each other. With your elbows straight and shoulders away from ears, rise into Dhanurasana.

- Ardha Dhanurasana (Half Bow Pose): Instead of holding both ankles, it's easier to do one side at a time. Prop yourself up on your right forearm, with the forearm perpendicular to your spine, upper arm vertical. Bend your left knee and grasp the ankle with the left hand. Proceed as above. Minimize the twist in the spine by reaching forward with the left side of the chest. Don't rest weight on your right elbow; rather, press up with the right

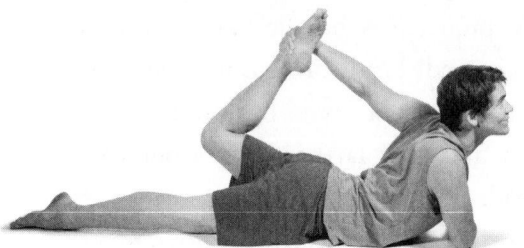

arm, and reach back and up with the left leg. To deepen the bend, engage your spinal muscles and pull lightly against the left leg with your left arm; don't overarch the lower spine. After you exit and pause in the prone position (head turned to one side), repeat on the other side.

Vasishthasana—Vasishtha's[8] Pose

Vasishthasana invigorates the entire body, especially the spine and trunk. See the asana not in terms of muscle endurance, but in terms of endurance of concentration on the energy that animates the muscles to support the body's straightness and length in this pose. When you add relaxation to your concentration, you'll gain an experience of powerful, focused stillness after the asana—and with practice, even while you're in the asana. Fan the flames of your ability to concentrate, affirming,

> *"The calm fire of my concentration burns all restlessness, all distraction."*

Technique

Begin in the Plank Pose: your body is in a straight line, resting on hands and toes, with hands beneath shoulders. Bring your feet together.

On an inhalation, transfer your upper body weight onto your left arm, sweep your right arm out to the side and up, and turn your body 90 degrees to the right, so that your right leg and foot rest atop the left.

---

[8] Vasishtha was an ancient Indian master of Yoga.

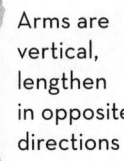

Arms are
vertical,
lengthen
in opposite
directions

Your body should still be in a straight line from the feet to the crown of the head—neither sagging toward the floor nor arching toward the sky. Your arms should be vertical, lengthening in opposite directions. Don't let your weight sink into your left shoulder; rather, lengthen up strongly through the left arm as it supports your weight.

Gaze straight ahead, or turn your head to gaze up past your right hand. Breathe smoothly and naturally, mentally affirming, *"The calm fire of my concentration burns all restlessness, all distraction."*

Exit gracefully to Balasana (Child Pose) or to a comfortable sitting position. Pause, then repeat on the other side.

Spine is
straight

Legs align with spine

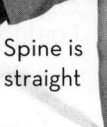

Variations

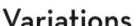

- Easier: If it's difficult to balance, bring the right foot forward onto the floor instead of resting it atop the left.
- Easier: Support your weight on the left forearm and left knee, with both knees bent 90 degrees and the right leg resting atop the left. Take extra care not to let your weight sink into your left shoulder.

Mayurasana—Peacock Pose

Mayurasana is extraordinarily vitalizing for the entire body and mind. It's fun to "fly," once you find a variation of Peacock Pose that works for you. Simply keep your body long, straight, and balanced—lengthening it with energy, not merely with muscle power. Concentrate on that lengthening energy, and enjoy the awakened energy itself as the asana's affirmation.

Technique

Kneel with your hands between your knees, palms on the floor with fingers pointing back toward your feet—hands close to each other. Spread your fingers wide. Bend your elbows to about 90 degrees, bring them directly over the hands (or nearly so), and lower your abdomen onto your elbows, with the spine straight.

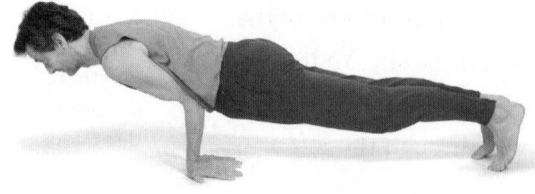

Step your feet back so that your body is supported on your hands and toes, and it's in a straight line from feet to crown of head. Most of your weight will now be on your elbows, which you should keep close together. Lift through the backs of your thighs. Gaze forward and slightly down, maintaining openness in the back of your neck. This position is Ardha Mayurasana (Half Peacock Pose).

For Full Peacock, slowly walk your feet forward until your legs lift off the floor and your entire weight is balanced on your hands. Keep lifting through the backs of your thighs. The body should now be horizontal. Gaze down and slightly forward.

Sustain that horizontal position by lengthening your body with energy, more than by holding it up with muscle strength. Breathe as smoothly as possible as you remain balanced, *but do breathe.* Let your experience of the vibrant energy of this pose—especially in your abdominal region and along the back of your body—be your asana affirmation.

Exit *gracefully* to Balasana (Child Pose) or to a comfortable sitting position, and pause.

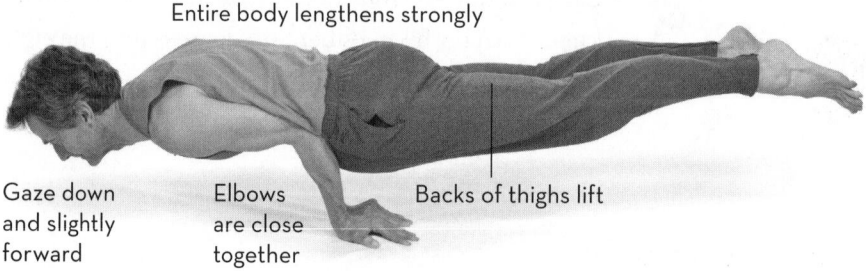

Entire body lengthens strongly

Gaze down and slightly forward   Elbows are close together   Backs of thighs lift

Variations

• Easier: If your torso slips between your elbows, make a loop with a strap, and place it around your upper arms near the elbows to keep the elbows closer together. If comfort dictates that your elbows be farther apart (e.g., a woman's breasts might be pressed uncomfortably when the elbows are close together and body weight is resting on the elbows), then separate the hands accordingly, again with a strap around the arms.

• Easier: From Ardha Mayurasana, bring your knees to the floor and bend them so that your feet come up behind you. You might feel more stable if you cross your ankles. Then proceed as above. You'll feel even more stable if you can bring your legs into Padmasana (Lotus Pose), because that locks the legs together. Padmasana itself is not easy, of course, but if you can do it, Padma Mayurasana (Lotus Peacock Pose) becomes easier than standard Mayurasana, because your body is more compact, which makes it easier both to balance and to hold the horizontal position.

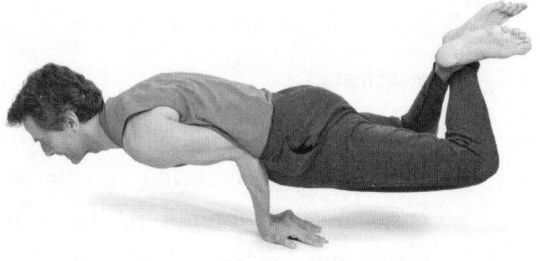

Simhasana—Lion Pose

Every facet of this pose—bodily posture and movement, breath and energy control, direction of the gaze, object of concentration, use of the will—helps to bring energy to the fifth chakra (bishuddha chakra in Sanskrit). This chakra is important for clear communication, for a connection between mind and heart, and above all, for experiencing the qualities of calmness and expansion of consciousness. The abundant energy in the throat will reinforce those qualities as you affirm,

"I purify my thoughts, my speech, my every action."

Technique

Sit in Vajrasana (Firm Pose) with palms on your knees, fingers spread wide. As energy rises up the spine with an inhalation, lift your chest. Then as you retain the breath, open your mouth and eyes wide; thrust your tongue out and down as far as possible, and gaze downward intensely. Lightly tense the entire body, as though you were a lion about to spring. The sense of springing, however, should be inward, with no thought of anything outward toward which to spring.

While retaining the breath, concentrate your energy and awareness in the throat, and silently repeat the affirmation: *"I purify my thoughts, my speech, my every action."*

Exhale when you need to, and repeat the above process with the next breath. Continue for as many breaths as you wish. Afterward, pause in Vajrasana.

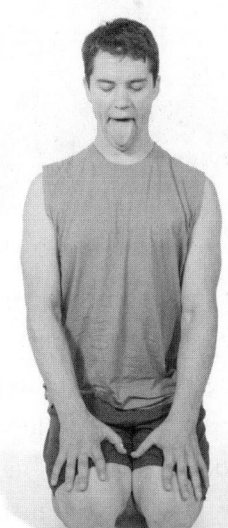

Tongue and gaze are directed downward

Energy and attention are focused in throat

Body is lightly tensed

Retain the breath

Variations

- Instead of resting the tops of the toes on the floor, curl your toes under. If this position is comfortable, it can bring a greater sense of aliveness to the asana.
- Easier: Instead of retaining the breath, let it flow naturally. Keep your chest lifted, tongue thrust out, and body lightly tensed. Gaze downward intently for the duration of the asana.
- For ankle or knee discomfort: Use props as described for Vajrasana.

Yoga Mudra—Symbol of Yoga

Yoga Mudra is the ultimate position of self-surrender: the deep forward bow fully exposes the medulla oblongata (seat of the ego); the hand mudra magnetically directs energy up the spine, through the medulla oblongata; and the gentle pressure of the forehead on the floor helps redirect your awareness (and thus your energy) to the spiritual eye. Add your devotion to the experience, offering yourself completely into the inner light of the spiritual eye as you affirm,

"I am Thine; receive me."

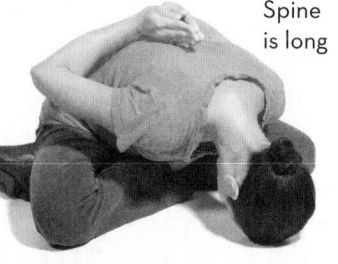

Pelvis rotates forward, sitbones grounded

Rotation is in hips, not knees or ankles

Spine is long

Knees are at or below hip level

Technique

Sit in a comfortable cross-legged position. Padmasana (Lotus Pose) is considered ideal; Swastikasana (Auspicious Pose) and Siddhasana (Perfect Pose) are also good options.

Join your palms *behind* you, fingers pointing upward along the spine.

Inhale and lengthen the spine, then exhale and bend forward from the hips as far as possible without rounding the spine. Then relax the spine and bring your forehead to the floor; keep as much length in the spine as possible. Close your eyes and gaze toward the spiritual eye.

Feel the combined influences of subtle gravity, the gentle pressure of the forehead resting on the floor, and the magnetism of your hands and fingers helping to bring your energies—especially those of the medulla oblongata—toward the spiritual eye. Add to those influences your own upward aspiration, your devotion. Breathe smoothly and naturally, silently affirming, *"I am Thine; receive me."*

To exit, inhale and return to upright, then release your hands to your lap, and pause.

Note: Because it brings energy directly to the spiritual eye, Yoga Mudra can also be highly beneficial right after deep relaxation in Savasana, before you meditate.

Variations

• Easier: If a cross-legged sitting position is uncomfortable, you can instead sit in Vajrasana, on a meditation bench, or on a chair. If you use a chair, place another chair in front of you, and rest your forehead on the seat of the second chair.
• Easier: If you're unable to join your palms behind you, then join your palms at the heart.
• Easier: If your forehead doesn't reach the floor, place a cushion in front of you, high enough that you can rest your forehead on it rather than let your head hang in the air.

Parvatasana—(Seated) Mountain Pose

The simplicity of Parvatasana masks its power: the breathing pattern lifts energy, the gentle abdominal bandha pushes energy upward from below, the upturned eyes direct energy upward, and the natural magnetism of the hand mudra attracts energy upward from above. Add one more element of power with your mind, as you affirm,

"My thoughts and energy rise up to touch the sky."

Technique

Sit in Padmasana (Lotus Pose) or any comfortable sitting position— on a cushion if needed to help you keep your spine straight.

On an inhalation, circle your hands out to the sides and up; join the palms overhead with the fingers pointing upward. As you exhale, relax your shoulders down and bend your elbows somewhat. Behind closed eyelids, lift your gaze toward the spiritual eye. Stay in this position throughout the asana.

As you finish your next inhalation, smoothly draw in your abdomen to focus energy in your upper torso (a firm, but gentle action). Keep your chest and shoulders open.

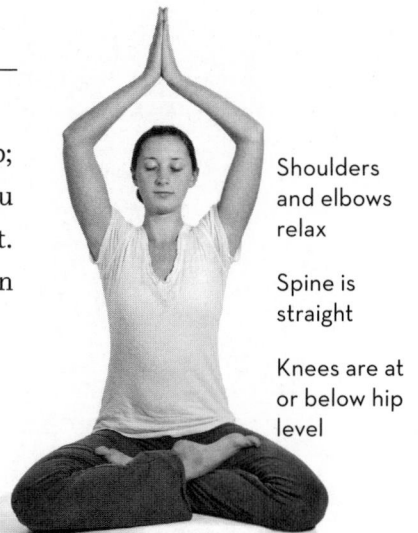

Shoulders and elbows relax

Spine is straight

Knees are at or below hip level

Knees and ankles are not strained

Retain the breath as long as comfortable, and mentally affirm, *"My thoughts and energy rise up to touch the sky."* Exhale when you need to.

Repeat this breathing pattern, bandha, and affirmation for as many breaths as you wish. Exit by returning to your original sitting position on an exhalation, and pause.

Note: Because Parvatasana lifts energy so effectively, it also can be highly beneficial right after deep relaxation in Savasana, before you meditate.

Variations

• Easier: If tight shoulders cause your hands to float in front of your body rather than overhead, or cause you to arch your spine into a backward bend, bend your elbows more to make it easier to have the hands overhead without arching. Alternatively, join the palms at the heart and use the natural magnetism of the hands and fingers to *direct* energy upward (as opposed to *attracting* energy upward, as in the standard asana).

4.5—INVERTED ASANAS: BRING ENERGY TO YOUR BRAIN

The highest purpose of Yoga is simply to place yourself in a position to receive fully a downpouring of Spirit. If God's grace is not experienced in the average human life, it is not because of divine indifference, but because man's energies and attention are diverted elsewhere.

—SWAMI KRIYANANDA

Your routine so far has helped you open the spine, and concentrate your energy and awareness there. It's probably also brought some energy to your brain, because many of the preceding asanas do that—especially partially inverted asanas such as Sasamgasana (Hare Pose) and Chakrasana (Wheel Pose), which ally somewhat with the force of subtle gravity. Now you'll ally more fully with subtle gravity to bring even more energy to your brain via the full inversions, i.e., asanas in which all, or almost all, of the spine is completely upside down.

Practice Tips

- Use props as needed for stability, safety, and neck comfort. For example, the first four inverted asanas below recommend lying on one or more folded blankets in order to cushion your vertebrae and to avoid overstretching your cervical spine (neck), which would make the neck more vulnerable to injury. To fold the average asana blanket (cotton Mexican blanket for a twin-sized bed), hold it completely open, one end in each hand, with the long dimension horizontal. Bring your hands together to fold the blanket horizontally, 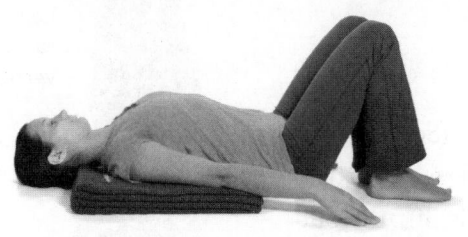 then fold it a second time vertically, then a third time horizontally. (A larger blanket might call for an additional fold or two.) Lie down with shoulders and arms on the blankets; the folded edges are under your neck, a few inches above your shoulders, and your head is on the floor.

- Don't sink onto your foundation. Use the body parts that touch the floor in the same way that you use your feet in standing asanas: as a firm foundation for stability, and as a point from which to lengthen up through your entire body. Press those parts into the floor—yes, press even the back of the head into the floor in such asanas as Sarvangasana

(Shoulderstand) and Halasana (Plow Pose)—and lengthen up through all parts of your body that are vertical; this will bring lightness, length, lifting, and life to the asana.

- Move slowly, with control. Flinging your body up into—or collapsing out of—an inverted asana can be jarring to your consciousness; it can also injure you.

- Don't depend on subtle gravity alone to bring energy to the brain. Use your feeling faculty to connect with energy, and your faculties of will and visualization to help move energy toward the brain. The asana descriptions offer tips for doing this.

- Let the body normalize after an inverted asana: stay down in Savasana (Corpse Pose) or Balasana (Child Pose) for a number of breaths before rising to an upright position. An immediate return to upright would agitate body and mind, and could cause a headache, dizziness, or even a fall.

Sarvangasana—Shoulderstand

Shoulderstand brings energy to the brain and exerts a peaceful, harmonizing influence on the entire body and mind. Attract those qualities to yourself by practicing in a spirit of peace and harmony. The more you do so, the more peace and harmony you'll receive. Hold the asana calmly and easily, lifting not only your body, but also your consciousness, like a chalice to receive the blessing of divine peace:

"God's peace now floods my being."

Technique

Lie on your back on two or more folded blankets. (See the first practice tip at the start of this section.) Lift your legs to vertical and, as you press down with your arms and hands, lift the buttocks and smoothly bring your knees over your face. Then reach your legs upward, straightening through your hip joints. Move with control, both for safety and for a deeper experience.

Place your hands on either side of your spine for support, as near to your shoulder blades as possible, with elbows shoulder-

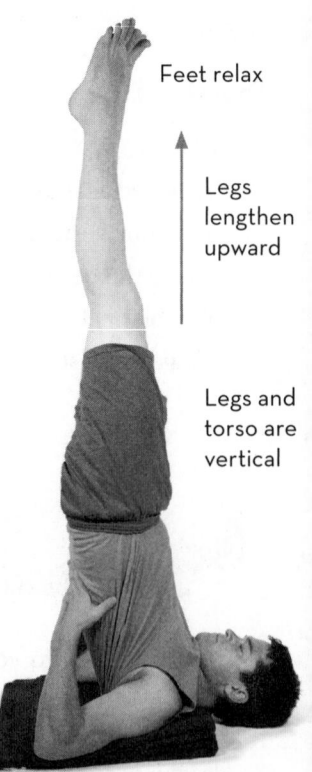

Feet relax

Legs lengthen upward

Legs and torso are vertical

Backs of arms, shoulders, and head press down

width apart. Roll your shoulders under, one at a time, and bring your legs and torso to vertical. Throughout the asana, press into the blankets with the backs of your arms and shoulders. Press into the floor with the back of your head to protect your neck from being overstretched as well as to keep the neck open so that energy can flow to the brain; don't turn your head.

Breathe smoothly and naturally, mentally affirming, *"God's peace now floods my being."*

To exit, bring your knees over your face, then release your hands to the floor, and use your arm and abdominal strength to control a slow return to the supine position. Remove the blankets and pause in Savasana (Corpse Pose).

Variation

• Easier (using a wall): Lie on the blankets with your buttocks at the wall, legs up the wall. Bend your knees if necessary to get your buttocks to the wall.

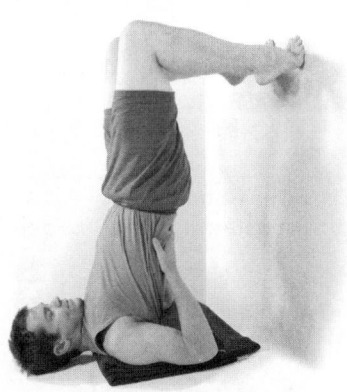

Bend your knees, place your feet flat on the wall, and press into the wall to lift the pelvis up and forward until torso and thighs are vertical. To reach vertical, you might need to walk your feet up or down the wall until your shins are horizontal; you might also need to come onto your toes.

Interlace your fingers and roll your shoulders under, one at a time. Unclasp your hands and place them on either side of the spine for support, as near to your shoulder blades as possible. Keep your elbows shoulder-width apart and press down with the backs of your arms, shoulders, and head.

Straighten one leg to vertical, away from the wall. Then straighten the other leg to enter the full pose. Alternatively, hold with one leg vertical for a time, then return it to the wall; repeat with the other leg.

To exit, bend your knees and bring your feet back to the wall, one at a time. Then slowly lower your pelvis to the floor. Pause with your legs up the wall, arms at your sides.

Viparita Karani—Simple Inverted Pose

In addition to being a full inversion, Viparita Karani takes advantage of the natural magnetism of your hands to stimulate and help release the Kundalini[9] energy that's trapped at the base of the spine. Then the force of subtle gravity—allied with your ability to feel and move energy—can draw that energy toward the brain. Use willpower and visualization to enhance this process, as you enthusiastically affirm,

"Awake, my sleeping powers, awake!"

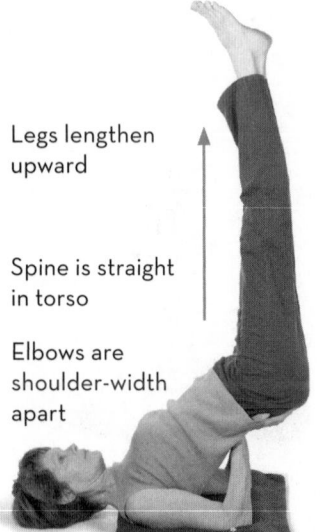

Legs lengthen upward

Spine is straight in torso

Elbows are shoulder-width apart

Backs of arms, shoulders, and head press down

Technique

Lie on your back (on a blanket if you wish; see the first practice tip at the start of this section). Lift your legs to vertical. Then, as you press down with your arms and hands, lift the buttocks and smoothly reach your legs upward. Move with control, both for safety and for a deeper experience.

Place the heels of your palms on the upper back rim of your pelvis, and roll your shoulders under, one at a time. Keep your elbows shoulder-width apart on the floor. Place your fingertips on the coccyx (tailbone). Your torso should be at about a 45-degree angle to the floor, and your legs should be vertical (or nearly vertical), so that a line straight down from your toes would intersect your abdomen.

Throughout the asana, press into the blanket/floor with the backs of your arms and shoulders. Press the back of your head into the floor as you lengthen upward through both legs; don't turn your head. To minimize wrist discomfort, press your fingers firmly against the coccyx.

Breathe smoothly and naturally, silently affirming, *"Awake, my sleeping powers, awake!"*

To exit, bring your knees over your face, then release your hands to the floor and use your arm and abdominal strength to control a slow return to the supine position. Remove the blanket and pause in Savasana (Corpse Pose).

---

9 Kundalini (literally, "the coiled") is a reservoir of energy at the base of the astral spine. It's the energetic result of the mindset that one is inherently separate from Spirit: emphasis on the small self traps energy at the base of the spine. Ego-centered thoughts and actions add to that reservoir, reinforcing one's feeling of separateness. Freeing some of that energy and moving it up the spine helps diminish the feeling and expand one's awareness. To reach the ultimate state of Self-realization, one must free all the Kundalini energy, and bring it up the spine to the brain.

Variations

• Easier: Use the wall as described for the Sarvangasana (Shoulderstand) variation on page 127.

• Easier: If the standard asana places too much weight on your arms and wrists, you can find some relief by bringing your toes over your face; you'll still receive most of the benefits of the asana. If, however, you need to bring your feet past your face, you'll lose the power of the asana, so instead practice at the wall; over time, you'll gradually gain the strength required to practice standard Viparita Karani.

Halasana—Plow Pose

Halasana stretches and opens the upper spine, and pours a strong current of energy into the brain—a current that can wash away old ways of thinking and being, and open you to new, more beneficial ways. Your results depend, not just on the power of subtle gravity, but on how much—and how magnetically—you open yourself to that current, as you affirm,

"New life, new consciousness now flood my brain!"

Technique

Lie on your back on two or more folded blankets. (See the first practice tip at the start of this section.) Raise your legs to vertical. Then, as you press down with your arms and hands, lift the buttocks and smoothly bring your legs over your face. Move with control, both for safety and for a deeper experience.

Sitbones reach upward

Legs lengthen out through heels

Spine is relatively straight in torso

Backs of arms, shoulders, and head press down

Slowly lower your toes to the floor beyond your head, with your legs and spine straight. Interlace your fingers behind you, and roll your shoulders under, one at a time, to enable you to straighten your spine and bring it to vertical. Throughout the asana, press into the blankets with your arms and shoulders to keep your spine relatively straight and vertical (except for the neck, of course). Press into the floor with the back of your head to protect your neck from being overstretched as well as to keep the neck open so that energy can flow to the brain; don't turn your head.

Breathe smoothly and naturally, silently affirming, *"New life, new consciousness now flood my brain!"*

To exit, lift your legs, separate your hands, and use your arm and abdominal strength to control a slow return to the supine position. Remove the blankets and pause in Savasana (Corpse Pose).

Variation

• Easier: If you're unable to bring your feet all the way to the floor while keeping your knees straight, rest your feet on a cushion, chair, or block behind you (anchored so as not to slide easily).

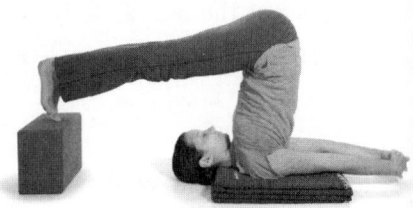

Karnapirasana—Ear-Closing Pose

Although visually similar to Halasana, Karnapirasana has quite different effects: whereas Halasana is dynamic, Karnapirasana is restful for both brain and body, bringing both into greater stillness. Entering Karnapirasana from Halasana can add vibrancy to that stillness. Take the stillness deeper by affirming,

"My boat of life floats lightly on tides of peace."

Technique

Lie on your back on two or more folded blankets. (See the first practice tip at the start of this section.) Raise your legs to vertical. Then, as you press down with your arms and hands, smoothly lift the buttocks and bring your legs over your face. Move with control, both for safety and for a deeper experience.

Keeping your spine long, allow your knees to bend and release toward the floor on either side of your head. It's fine for the spine to round somewhat, provided it feels comfortable and you're not forcing it to round. Lower your feet to the floor, with the tops of the feet (rather than the tips of the toes) resting on the floor.

Interlace your fingers behind you, and roll

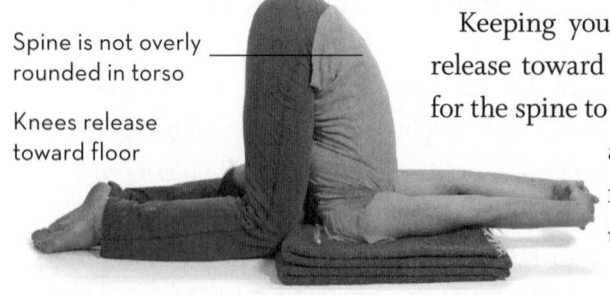

Spine is not overly rounded in torso

Knees release toward floor

Backs of arms, shoulders, and head press down

your shoulders under, one at a time, to enable your spine to be straighter and more vertical. Press the backs of your shoulders and arms into the floor to keep your spine long as you continue to relax your knees toward the floor. Press into the floor with the back of your head to protect your neck from being overstretched as well as to keep the neck open so that energy can flow to the brain; don't turn your head.

Breathe smoothly and naturally, mentally affirming, *"My boat of life floats lightly on tides of peace."*

To exit, lift your legs, separate your hands, and use your arm and abdominal strength to control a slow return to the supine position. Remove the blankets and pause in Savasana (Corpse Pose).

Variations

- Easier: If you're unable to bring your feet all the way to the floor while keeping your knees straight, rest the tops of your feet on a cushion behind you.
- More advanced: To deepen both the upper spinal stretch and your inner silence, place your palms over your ears, with the backs of the hands against the inner knees.

Sirshasana—Headstand

Here is the supreme inversion: with the body totally upside down, the force of subtle gravity can easily draw abundant energy to the brain. Use your faculties of willpower and visualization, plus a joyful attitude, to increase that flow and focus it at the point between the eyebrows. This will invigorate your higher functions—creativity, joy, concentration, spiritual insight, willpower, and more—so that you may move toward the perception of your own divine essence. Aid the process by affirming that essence,

"I am He! I am He! Blissful Spirit, I am He!"

Technique

CAUTION: Sirshasana is not for beginners. Before you try the full asana, master the easier variations given below until you develop the strength to remain stable and avoid straining your neck.

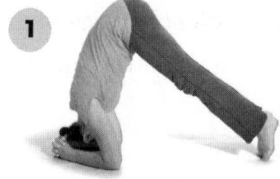

Kneel with your forearms on the floor in front of you, elbows shoulder-width apart and fingers interlaced. Place the crown of your head on the floor, and cradle the back of your head in the pocket formed by your hands.

Phase 1: Turn your toes under, lift your knees, and walk your feet toward your head until your torso is vertical (or nearly so); your weight will now be primarily on your forearms and elbows. Stabilize your shoulders by drawing the upper arm bones into their shoulder sockets and pressing down through the elbows. Throughout the asana, press down strongly with your shoulders, keep your spine straight and shoulders as far from the floor as possible, and rest only minimal weight on the crown of your head.

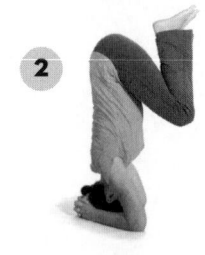

Phase 2: Bend your knees and walk your feet closer until your thighs are against your torso. Now shift all your weight onto your arms and head—almost all the weight is on your arms—and slowly bend your knees even more to lift your feet off the floor. Pause here to stabilize your position and ensure that your spine is straight before proceeding.

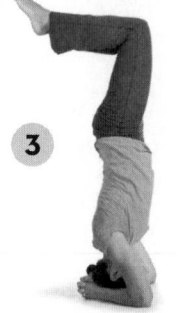

Phase 3: Keep your knees bent as you straighten your hips until your thighs are vertical.

Phase 4: Straighten your knees into the completed asana, and lengthen up through the legs. The gentle pressure of the crown of your head on the floor helps redirect your awareness (and therefore your energy) to the brain, and subtle gravity will pull energy to the brain. Bring even more energy to the brain through willpower, visualization, and a joyful attitude. Concentrate that energy at the spiritual eye.

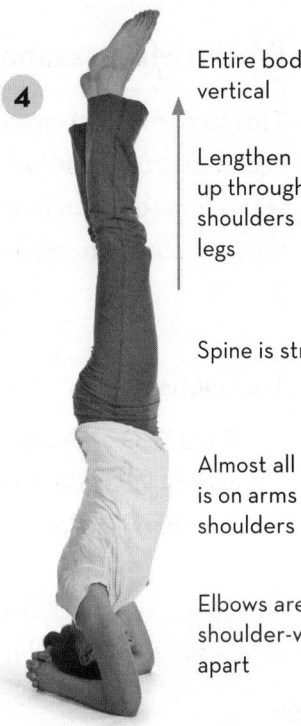

4

Entire body is vertical

Lengthen up through shoulders and legs

Spine is straight

Almost all weight is on arms and shoulders

Elbows are shoulder-width apart

Breathe smoothly and naturally, silently affirming the ultimate truth of your being: *"I am He! I am He! Blissful Spirit, I am He!"*

Stay in the asana only as long as you're able to support most of your weight on your forearms and elbows.

To exit, reverse the steps: Fold your knees, then fold your hips, then relax your toes to the floor. Transfer weight onto your legs, soften your knees to the floor, and pause in Balasana (Child Pose).

Variations

• Easier: Rather than going into the full asana, stay in Phase 1 (or 2, or 3) to practice your balance and to become better able to support your weight primarily with shoulder strength rather than by resting substantial weight on your head and neck.

• Easier: From Phase 1, lift your feet one at a time onto a stable platform (a chair seat or a large block, anchored so as to be stable). Holding this position will strengthen your shoulders as well as give you many of the benefits of the full asana. If you feel secure in this position, lift one leg as high as you can, with the other foot still on the chair. Hold for a time, then bring the leg back down. Repeat with the other leg.

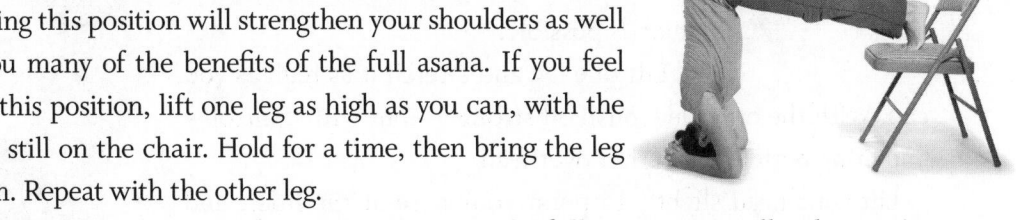

• Easier: For extra support and safety when practicing the full pose—especially when you're first learning the full pose—do Sirshasana with the back of your body against a wall, or better still, in the corner of a room, so that you could not fall backwards or sideways.

Pincha Mayurasana—Peacock Feather Pose

This forearm balance isn't just acrobatics: it combines a full inversion with an energizing backward bend, without strain on your cervical spine (neck). As you hold the asana, open yourself to the abundant life-force pouring through the spine to your spiritual eye, reinforcing your resolve to realize the highest that is within you:

"The Infinite Light cascades through my spine."

Technique

CAUTION: Pincha Mayurasana is not for beginners. Before you try the full asana, master the easier variations given below until you develop the shoulder strength and shoulder flexibility necessary for the full asana.

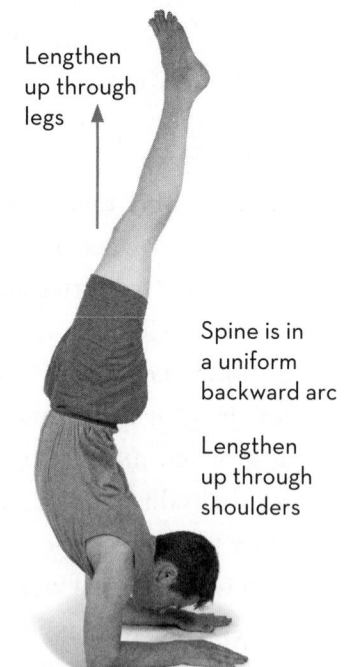

Lengthen up through legs

Spine is in a uniform backward arc

Lengthen up through shoulders

Hands and elbows are shoulder-width apart

Come onto your forearms and knees, with elbows and hands shoulder-width apart.

Straighten your spine, draw your upper arm bones into the shoulder sockets to stabilize the shoulders, and press down through the elbows. Lift your knees off the floor and walk your toes forward, to bring your torso closer to vertical. Throughout the asana, press down strongly with your shoulders and keep them as far from the floor as possible.

Lift one leg and stretch it as high as you can. With the other leg, push off strongly—but with control—and bring both legs together overhead.

Lift your head slightly to point your nose at the floor, and gaze toward the spiritual eye. Stabilize your body by pressing down through the shoulders.

Your entire body (from feet to head) will now be in a graceful backward bend. If the weight of your legs causes your lower spine to overarch, then reach up more strongly through the legs and/or draw your navel toward the spine to flatten the arch a bit.

Breathe smoothly and naturally, mentally affirming, *"The Infinite Light cascades through my spine."*

To exit, bring one leg down, then the other, and pause in Balasana (Child Pose).

Variations

- Easier: If your elbows splay out to the sides, tie a strap around the upper arms, just above the elbows. Or place a book or block inside the "L" shape between the widespread thumbs and forefingers.
- Easier: From the forearms and knees position, lift your feet one at a time onto a stable platform (a chair seat or a large block, anchored so as to be stable). Holding this position will strengthen your shoulders until they can support your entire body weight; attempting Pincha Mayurasana without sufficient shoulder strength or shoulder flexibility can injure your shoulders or cause a fall. Practicing this variation is the safest way to begin learning Pincha Mayurasana. If you feel secure in this position, lift one leg as high as you can, with the other foot still on the chair. Hold for a time, then bring the leg back down. Repeat with the other leg.
- Easier: For extra support and safety when practicing the full pose—especially when you're first learning the full pose—do Pincha Mayurasana with your back to a wall. Place your fingertips at the base of the wall. Your heels will rest against the wall when you come up into the asana.

4.6—RELAXATION ASANAS: RELAX ON ALL LEVELS

It is impossible to develop true Self-awareness without first learning how to relax. Energy that is bound cannot soar to divine heights. The science of Yoga might even be defined as a process of progressive relaxation: first, from outer attachments; then from attachment to body, to thoughts, to personality, to ego—until you find yourself at last in the stream of infinite life.

—SWAMI KRIYANANDA

Relaxation is important in all asanas, even in those that require a lot of physical effort. The two asanas in this section, however, call for the absence not only of physical effort, but also of all physical tension—even tension that you're holding unconsciously. These physical aspects of relaxation can be challenging enough in themselves. Complete relaxation, however, as Kriyananda emphasizes in the above quotation, comes only with relaxation on levels *beyond* the physical level. Here are some tips to help you do that:

Practice Tips

- Begin with the "hot spots": consciously relax the places where you habitually hold tension, as well as any body parts that were working hard in the preceding asana(s). One way to do so is to tense and relax in those places several times.
- Breathe slowly and naturally. With each exhalation, feel a sense of withdrawal: energy withdrawing from body parts that were working hard, as well as withdrawal of your awareness from outer involvements, body attachment, worries, regrets, thoughts, and desires—toward the one true reality of divine consciousness.
- Lift your gaze toward the spiritual eye. When most people relax, past habit tends to take them toward the subconscious state of sleep, in which the eyes ordinarily turn downward. Therefore keep your eyes turned upward, behind closed eyelids—not merely to help you stay awake, but to help you cultivate superconscious relaxation.
- Give a direction to your relaxation: inward from your periphery to the spine, and upward toward the spiritual eye.

Balasana—Child Pose

Balasana naturally—almost automatically—calms and internalizes your awareness. Use whatever props you need in order to relax more fully, and thereby receive these benefits. Stay alert by lifting your gaze toward the spiritual eye; then you can more easily relax energy and awareness from your periphery into your center, as you affirm,

"I relax from outer involvement into my inner haven of peace."

Technique

From Vajrasana (Firm Pose), release your hands to your sides. Inhale and lengthen your spine, then as you exhale, bend forward from the hips and bring your forehead to the floor. Rest your hands on the floor by your feet, palms facing up.

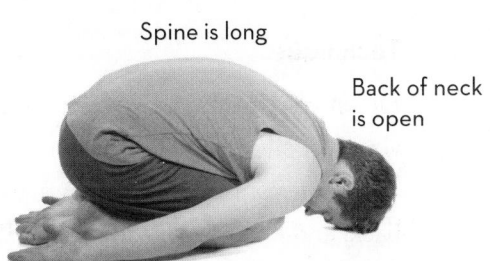

Spine is long

Back of neck is open

Entire body is relaxed

Relax your body completely, and breathe smoothly and naturally; feel the breath massaging your abdomen and opening your back and shoulders.

Silently affirm, *"I relax from outer involvement into my inner haven of peace."*

To exit, inhale as you bring your torso slowly upright into Vajrasana.

Variations

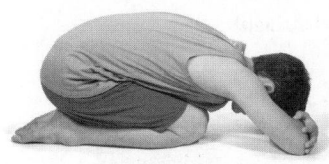

- For neck discomfort: Lengthen the back of your neck by bringing your chin closer to your chest, or by propping yourself up a bit on your elbows, holding opposite elbows, and resting your forehead on your forearms.
- For knee discomfort: Place a cushion between the buttocks and the backs of your ankles. Or separate your legs and sit on a tall cushion placed between the legs.
- For ankle discomfort: Place a rolled towel or rolled blanket under the fronts of your ankles.

Savasana—Corpse Pose

Practiced perfectly, Savasana brings relaxation on every level of your being. It also helps develop the deep receptivity that's vital to all of Yoga. Although perfect relaxation can be elusive, Savasana's affirmation is a great aid. Move slowly through its phrases, consciously letting go on each level—physical, then emotional, then mental, and finally spiritual—before moving to the next:

> *"Bones, muscles, movement I surrender now; anxiety, elation and
> depression, churning thoughts—all these I give into the hands of peace."*

Technique

Lie on your back and stretch your legs away from your head to lengthen your spine. Rest your feet slightly wider than hip-width apart; let them roll out to the sides.

Stretch your shoulders down away from your ears; slide your shoulder blades down your back, and keep them wide apart. Rest your arms near your sides, but far enough away from your body to maintain an open feeling in your armpits. Turn your inner arms and palms upward. Lengthen through the back of your neck, bringing ears away from shoulders. Your entire spine should be neutral. (For people with bulky shoulders, this might require placing a small cushion under the head.)

With eyes closed, lift your gaze toward the spiritual eye.

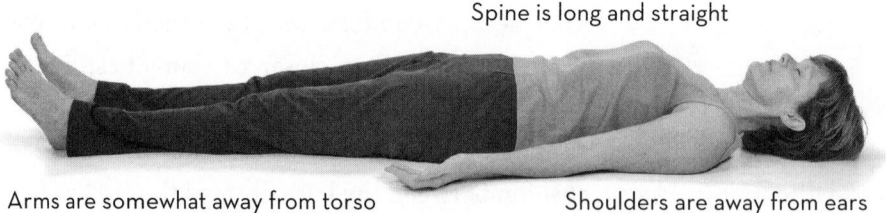

Spine is long and straight

Arms are somewhat away from torso   Shoulders are away from ears

Savasana Between Two Active Asanas

Lie in the above position until any energy stirred up by the preceding asana has become calm once again, or, if the preceding asana was an inverted asana, until your body has normalized enough that's okay to come upright. If you were challenging a particular part of the body in the preceding asana—stretching it, or perhaps working it hard—focus first on relaxing that body part, then turn to relaxing the entire body.

After a brief pause in Savasana, move to the next active asana.

Savasana as Deep Relaxation

For a deeper level of relaxation, you'll need to relax not only tensions that you're aware of, but also tensions that lurk beneath your conscious level of awareness. One way to do so is to inhale, then tense the whole body as you retain the breath. Then exhale and relax the entire body. Repeat 2–3 times; use a Double Breath (see Section 5.2) if you like.

Next, let go of the breath and simply notice it as it flows in and out through the nostrils. As your mind becomes calmer and your breath becomes quieter, feel your consciousness becoming centered increasingly, naturally, at the point between the eyebrows.

Now strive for *deep* relaxation. Feel your body surrounded by infinite space in all directions. Visualize this space seeping through the pores of the skin into your feet, until your feet *become* space. Slowly move up through the body, each part in turn becoming space: calves, thighs, hips, lower abdomen, lower back, upper abdomen, hands, forearms, upper arms, shoulders, chest, neck, jaw, tongue, lips, cheeks, eyes, ears, scalp, and brain.

Release into that infinite space any regrets about the past, any worries about the future. Let them dissipate in infinity. Rest in the perfection of the eternal Present. Nothing exists but this moment, and the soothing, loving divine presence that permeates this moment. Affirm mentally, *"Bones, muscles, movement I surrender now; anxiety, elation and depression, churning thoughts—all these I give into the hands of peace."*

Remain in stillness as long as you wish, with your gaze lifted toward the spiritual eye; immerse your entire being in divine peace.

Before returning to an upright sitting position, slowly and gently move your various body parts to bring them back to your awareness. Then bring your knees up, squeeze them into the torso, and roll left and right across your spine a few times. Roll over onto your right side, and stay there for several breaths. Then slowly bring yourself upright by pressing into the floor with your left hand and right elbow.

Variations

- For low back discomfort: Place a cushion or a rolled blanket under your knees.
- For bulky shoulders: If your neck is not in line with the rest of your spine (i.e., your head drops back sharply to the floor), place a small cushion under your head to straighten your neck.

4.7—SITTING ASANAS: INTERNALIZE YOUR AWARENESS

In meditation, try to raise your energy and consciousness up through the spine to the point between the eyebrows. This principle should also be followed during the practice of yoga postures. Seek by means of these postures to direct the body's energy up toward the brain. Do not allow it to become wasted in physical or mental tension, or in restless movements.

—SWAMI KRIYANANDA

Having completed your other asanas—having, that is, brought abundant energy inward from your periphery and upward to the brain—it's time to use that energy for pranayama, and especially meditation. The asanas in this section are ideal for this purpose: yogis say that these asanas help induce physical and mental steadiness by exerting a beneficial pressure on certain nerves, and that because the feet are upturned, close to the body, it's easier to raise your consciousness (the soles of the feet are sensitive energy receptors). These asanas also can be used as neutral asanas between active floor asanas.

Practice Tips

- Keep your spine straight. That will be easier if you sit with your knees slightly lower than your hips. To do this in a cross-legged asana, you might need to sit on a cushion, with your sitbones on the front edge of the cushion.
- Know your limits. You could injure your knees or ankles if you try to force your legs into some of these asanas before your hips are loose enough. It may take months, even years, of stretching to attain that degree of flexibility, so be patient.
- If either knee floats off the floor in a cross-legged asana, place a cushion under it without lifting the knee higher.
- A yogi need not sit in any of these asanas—ever! Yes, for meditation it's considered ideal to sit on the floor (usually cross-legged), but it's not vital. So if you find all these sitting asanas uncomfortable, even with props, then sit on a chair or a meditation bench (see Section 6.1). You can still attain the highest levels of consciousness.

Sukhasana—Easy Pose

Sukhasana is the simple tailor position of crossed legs. It's fine as a brief pause in a neutral pose. If you want to sit for a longer period—as when practicing pranayama or meditation—you can use props as described below, but if one of the other sitting asanas is comfortable for you, that's a better option.

Technique

Sit with knees bent and feet flat on the floor. Relax your knees out to the sides, with your right foot under your outer left calf, and your left foot under your outer right calf. Let both legs relax. Because the feet are underneath the lower legs, the knees will be off the floor, higher than your hips. That's okay for a brief period, but if you intend to sit for longer (such as for pranayama or meditation), sit on one or more cushions in order to make the knees lower than the hips and thereby make it feasible to maintain a straight spine for a longer time; or better still, choose one of the other sitting asanas.

Place your hands on your thighs, palms up, where the thighs meet the abdomen. Open your chest and relax your shoulders. Close your eyes and lift your gaze toward the point between the eyebrows.

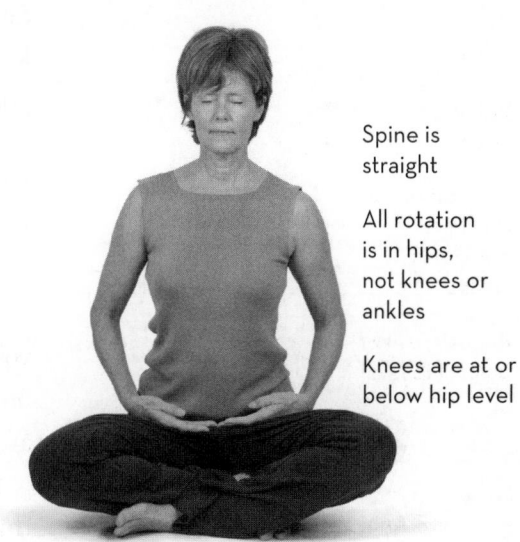

Spine is straight

All rotation is in hips, not knees or ankles

Knees are at or below hip level

Knees and ankles are not strained

Variation

• If practicing Sukhasana regularly, interchange the leg positions occasionally, so that your hips will stretch symmetrically over time.

Swastikasana—Auspicious Pose

Because the legs are somewhat locked together, this cross-legged position offers more stability than Sukhasana; it's also easier to position the knees lower than the hips, which helps you sit with a straight spine. These factors—plus the fact that it's a relatively easy asana—make Swastikasana an excellent option for pranayama and meditation.

Technique

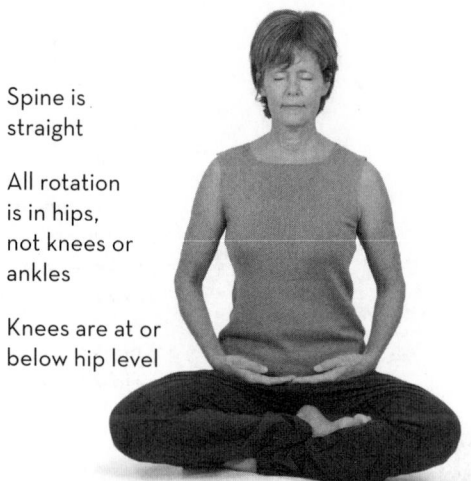

Spine is straight

All rotation is in hips, not knees or ankles

Knees are at or below hip level

Knees and ankles are not strained

Sit with knees bent and feet flat on the floor. Relax your knees out to the sides. Place the left foot under the crease between right thigh and calf, and relax the left knee to the floor. Rest the right foot atop the crease between the left thigh and calf. Be careful not to twist either knee as you assume the position. Rest the right knee on the floor if possible; if it's uncomfortably off the floor, place a cushion under it without raising the knee farther. If you're sitting for a longer period, you'll likely need to sit on the front edge of a cushion to ensure that your knees are lower than your hips and your spine stays straight.

Place your hands on your thighs, palms up, where the thighs meet the abdomen. Open your chest and relax your shoulders. Close your eyes and lift your gaze toward the point between the eyebrows.

Variation

• If practicing Swastikasana regularly—especially if you hold it for longer periods of time—interchange the leg positions occasionally, so that your hips will stretch symmetrically over time.

Vajrasana—Firm Pose (aka Thunderbolt Pose)

In Firm Pose, the weight of the upper body on the legs suggests to the mind a sense of bodily heaviness, of the body sinking away from your awareness. This is one of the few asanas in which such a sense of heaviness can be helpful, for then the mind is naturally drawn to function on levels subtler than the physical: you become more aware of the inner energies that move freely even while the physical body is still. Identify more and more with those energies—less and less with the physical body—as your reality:

"In stillness I touch my inner strength."

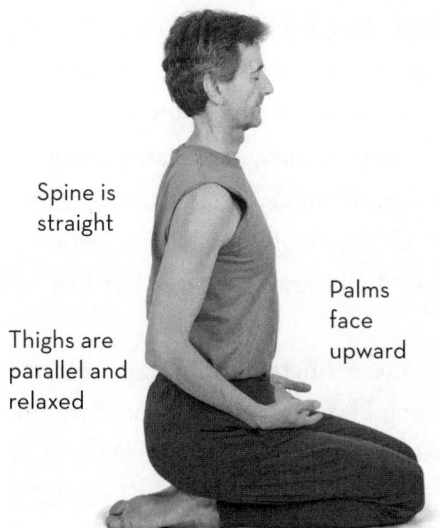

Spine is straight

Thighs are parallel and relaxed

Palms face upward

Right big toe covers left big toe

Technique

Sit on your heels, with your thighs parallel and toes pointing behind you. Cross your right big toe over your left big toe (provided that's comfortable for you), and relax your legs completely.

Place your hands on your thighs, palms up, where the thighs meet the abdomen. Leave your legs relaxed as you lengthen your spine, open your chest, and relax your shoulders. Close your eyes and lift your gaze toward the spiritual eye.

Breathe smoothly and naturally, mentally affirming, *"In stillness I touch my inner strength."*

Variations

- For knee discomfort: Place a cushion between the buttocks and the backs of your ankles. Or separate your legs, and sit on a tall cushion placed between the legs. Or sit on a meditation bench (see Section 6.1).
- For ankle discomfort: Place a rolled blanket or rolled towel under the fronts of your ankles.

Siddhasana—Perfect Pose

In Perfect Pose, your body becomes very stable because your legs are locked in place. With the heels pressing close to the base of the spine, energy is pushed from the lower extremities to the base of the spine, then up toward the brain, thereby helping to raise your awareness. To enhance this effect, strive to help move the energy upward by applying your inner faculties of energy-awareness, will, and visualization—all aided by a joyful attitude—as you affirm,

"I set ablaze the fire of inner joy."

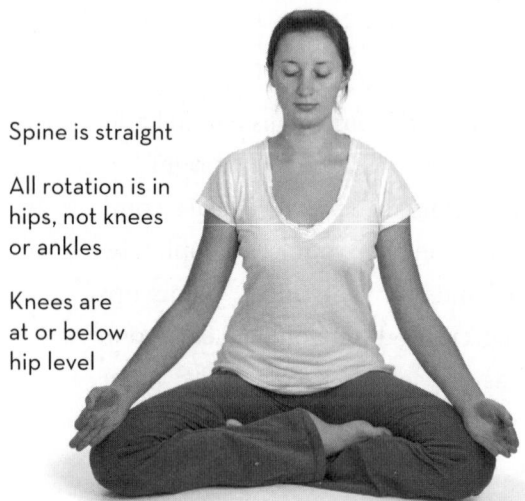

Spine is straight

All rotation is in hips, not knees or ankles

Knees are at or below hip level

Knees and ankles are not strained

Technique

Sit with knees bent, feet flat on the floor. Rotating from your left hip joint, release your left knee onto the floor, and slide your left heel into your groin.

Do the same with your right knee, and rest your right ankle atop the left ankle. Tuck your right foot between your left calf and thigh. Reach down between your right calf and thigh, and pull your left foot up between them.

If your ankles press uncomfortably against one another, put padding between them. If you have difficulty keeping a straight spine, sit on the front edge of a cushion. Place a cushion under the right knee if it's significantly off the floor.

Rest your hands on your thighs near your knees, palms facing up, in Gyana Mudra (Symbol of Wisdom): make a circle by joining the tips of the thumb and forefinger of each hand; extend the other three fingers. Lengthen your spine, open your chest, and relax your shoulders. Close your eyes and lift your gaze toward the spiritual eye.

Feel how the body position facilitates both stability and an upward push on the spinal energies. Breathe smoothly and naturally, and cooperate with that upward push by silently affirming, *"I set ablaze the fire of inner joy."*

Variations

• Easier (Ardha Siddhasana, Half Perfect Pose): Same as above except that your right foot stays on the floor, in front of your left foot.
• If doing Siddhasana or Ardha Siddhasana regularly, interchange the leg positions occasionally so that your hips will stretch symmetrically over time.

Padmasana—Lotus Pose

This is the ideal position for pranayama and meditation. Its every aspect promotes a natural rising of energy and consciousness: physical stability (the legs are locked together physically), the upturned palms of the hands and soles of the feet (these are sensitive energy receptors), straight spine, uplifted gaze. Add your powers of calm enthusiasm, visualization, and joyful self-offering, affirming:

"I sit serene, uplifted in Thy light."

Technique

CAUTION: Most people need months, even years, of stretching the muscles around the hips in order to practice Lotus Pose in a way that is safe for the knees and ankles. Be patient if you wish to work toward this asana, and remember: Hatha Yoga offers plenty of other ways to sit.

For knee and ankle safety when entering Padmasana, the movements of the legs should result primarily from action in the hip joints rather than in the knees or ankles. Also, keep your spine upright and straight while entering and holding Padmasana.

Sit upright with your legs straight in front of you. Bend your right knee and slide your right foot next to your left thigh, then rotate the right hip joint to bring your right knee onto (or near) the floor. Relax the right hip and, with both hands, lift your right leg and further rotate the right hip joint. Then move the leg to the left and place your right foot on your left thigh, near the hip crease. Press the little-toe side of the right foot into your left thigh to keep from sickling the foot (i.e., to keep the ankle from turning sideways significantly).

Bend your left knee and slide the left foot in toward you, then rotate your left hip joint to bring the left knee onto (or near) the floor. With both hands, lift your left leg and further rotate the left hip joint; keep both legs relaxed. When the left leg is sufficiently above the right, move it to the right and place the left foot on the right thigh, near the hip crease. Press the little-toe side of the left foot into the right thigh.

If it's difficult to keep your spine straight when entering or holding Padmasana, sit on the front edge of a cushion. If either knee is significantly off the floor, it would be best to spend more time stretching out your hips before attempting this pose.

Place your hands on your thighs, palms up, where the thighs meet the abdomen. Lengthen your spine, open your chest, and relax your shoulders. Close your eyes and lift your gaze toward the spiritual eye.

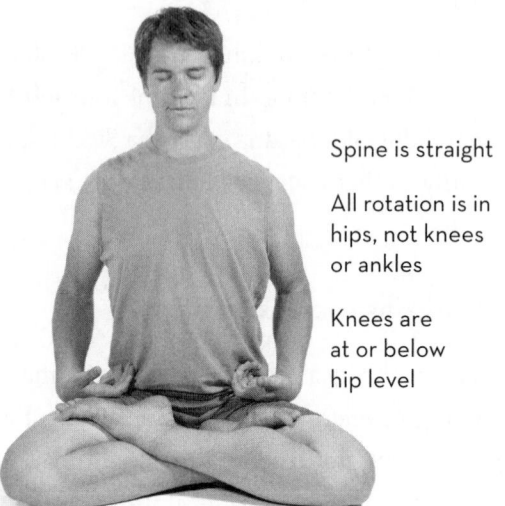

Spine is straight

All rotation is in hips, not knees or ankles

Knees are at or below hip level

Knees and ankles are not strained

Breathe smoothly and naturally, mentally affirming, "I sit serene, uplifted in Thy light."

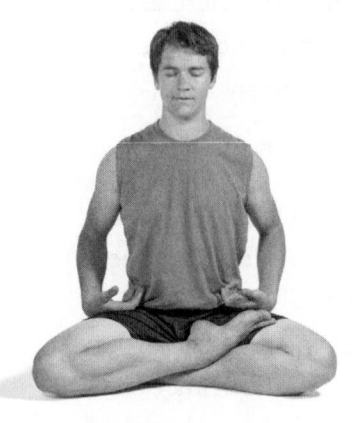

Variations

• Easier (Ardha Padmasana, Half Lotus Pose): Instead of crossing the left leg over the right, leave the left foot on the floor and place it under the right leg.

• If doing Padmasana or Ardha Padmasana regularly, interchange the leg positions occasionally so that your hips will stretch symmetrically over time.

Chapter
FIVE

Pranayamas

Transcendence is the goal of life. Rest is the goal of action.
Breathlessness is the final goal of all breathing exercises.
Breathlessness is deathlessness.

—SWAMI KRIYANANDA

To most people, breathlessness means, "I can't breathe." To the yogi, however, it means, "I don't *need* to breathe." It's a doorway to higher awareness, for just as the wind ruffles the surface of a lake, distorting the reflection of the moon overhead, so also the breath ruffles the mind, preventing one from seeing oneself as the perfect reflection of Spirit.

Pranayama (yogic breath-control) is one way to reach the breathless state. You won't get there by holding the breath forcibly, an approach that Paramhansa Yogananda described as "unscientific" and "not only unnatural, but decidedly unpleasant." No, that won't raise your consciousness. Instead, pranayama practice calls for sensitively controlling the breath, "shaping" the breath rather than being forceful. This will gradually and naturally calm the breath, heart, and mind; it might even relieve the body of its need to breathe at all, thereby freeing you to soar in superconsciousness.

Fortunately, you don't have to be in the breathless state in order to raise your consciousness. (What a relief!) Just as your bodily position can help you raise energy to the brain, so also can your breath. In fact, energy rises toward the brain every time you inhale; it also descends every time you exhale. As I noted in Chapter 1, those movements of energy naturally affect your state of mind.

Ordinary breaths don't impact your state of mind very much—thank goodness, else every breath would be a roller coaster ride!—but certain breathing patterns, sustained with focused intention, *can* have an impact. For example, a series of strong inhalations can energize you, make you more alert, and even uplift your state of mind; if you continue for too long, they can agitate you. Repeated strong exhalations can calm you; if you continue for too long, they can depress you, or at least dampen your enthusiasm. Smooth, deep, regular breathing helps relax you and reduce tension, anxiety, and stress; shallow, rapid, and/or irregular breathing can induce those undesirable states.

This breath-energy-mind connection is central to the effectiveness of Hatha Yoga's many different pranayamas. Each one helps you control energy in its own specific way. Greater control over energy will help you calm the heart, banish moods, uplift your state of mind, and move toward the breathless state, the deep inner stillness in which you can perceive the peace of the soul.

5.1—GUIDELINES FOR PRANAYAMA PRACTICE

The following guidelines apply to all the pranayamas, except where noted:

Sit Upright

For the deepest experience—and an effortless transition into meditation—sit upright with your spine straight, body relaxed, eyes closed and gaze lifted toward the spiritual eye. You can use a sitting asana (see Section 4.7), or a chair, or a meditation bench, which is almost the same as sitting in Vajrasana (Firm Pose). Place your hands on your thighs, palms up, where the thighs meet the abdomen. See Section 6.1 for more details on these sitting options.

Use Proper Breathing Mechanics

The effectiveness of all pranayamas depends on good breathing mechanics. Breathe naturally: the belly expands as you inhale, and relaxes back in as you exhale. If this breathing pattern isn't already a habit for you, your first step in pranayama is to make it so.

Breathe through your nose, not through your mouth. (There are exceptions: to achieve certain results, a few of the techniques below call for breathing through the mouth.) Nostril breathing filters out dust and other impurities that would otherwise enter the lungs; it also warms and moistens the air before it reaches the delicate inner membranes of the respiratory tract. On a deeper level, air coming in via the nasal passages cools, calms, and refreshes the brain; you'll think more clearly than when you breathe through your mouth.

Use Equal Inhalations and Exhalations

This helps balance the ascending and descending currents of energy in the spine, which is essential for attaining higher states of awareness. A few pranayama techniques call for unequal inhalations and exhalations for such special purposes as physical or emotional cleansing, or overcoming anxiety, depression, or insomnia. For spiritual purposes, however, equal is best, so that's what I'll present here. As you gain experience with these techniques, lengthen your inhalations and exhalations, but always keep them equal and free of strain.

One way to ensure equality is to count mentally as you inhale and exhale. This will also help you stay focused on the breath. Use whatever count is right for you: 4, 6, 8, or more.

Retain the Breath Comfortably

Many of these pranayamas call for retaining (holding) the breath: internally (after an inhalation) or externally (after an exhalation). Start with a period of internal retention equal to the length of the inhalations and exhalations; then lengthen it as you gain experience. Never strain; only through relaxation, concentration, and internalized awareness can you find such deep inner quiet that your mind will open naturally to higher states of awareness.

I'll focus mostly on internal retention, as it's easier for most people. External retention is a more advanced practice; it can be awkward at first, even agitating. Once internal retention feels natural, you can if you wish add external retention, which can quiet the breath and mind even more than can internal retention. Breathlessness itself is a state of effortless external retention. Also, affirmation is most effective during external retention.

Cultivate Breathlessness

Yes, cultivate longer inhalations, exhalations, and retentions—but that's not the goal of the practice; it's only a means to the goal: breathlessness and the resulting inner quiet that fosters deep meditation.

Therefore practice pranayama in such a way that every breath is an aid to quieting the mind: Breathe smoothly and evenly, with full attention. Follow the instructions, but try to go deeper, into the natural, intuitive flow of each technique. Never force the breath, but rather be sensitive to its reality, and cooperate with it. Notice the effect of the practice on your state of mind, and adjust—or even stop—if your mind becomes agitated. Realize that, because your body and mind change from day to day, your practice needs to vary as well: sometimes *this* technique is best, sometimes *that* one; sometimes longer inhalations and exhalations are better, sometimes shorter; sometimes it's a day for longer retentions, sometimes not.

Keep It Simple

It's not necessary, or even desirable, to practice all of Hatha Yoga's pranayamas. It's far better to do one or two deeply, attuning yourself sensitively to the flow of the astral (energy) breath; that's when you'll receive the greatest benefit.

Don't practice too many different pranayamas at one sitting, because depth of practice is superior to mere variety: one to three techniques is plenty. Also, choose techniques that take you in compatible, not conflicting, directions. For example, don't practice a stimulating technique such as Surya Bheda Pranayama (Expanding Sun Breath) immediately before or after a calming technique such as Sitali Pranayama (Cooling Breath). In fact, it's usually best not to practice conflicting pranayamas within the same routine—at least not a substantial period of both; a few minutes of each is okay if you have reason to do so, but space those periods well apart.

Equalize the Openness of Your Nostrils

At any given time, it's natural for one nostril to be dominant, i.e., more open than the other nostril. Nostril dominance switches sides every 90–120 minutes. However, in pranayama practice—especially in techniques that employ Vishnu Mudra (see Section 5.3)—it's ideal for the two nostrils to be equally open; this has to do with ease of breathing as well as raising consciousness. Unless you have sinus congestion, you can usually equalize the flow of breath by lying for 30–60 seconds on the side of your body corresponding to the dominant nostril.

How Long to Practice Pranayama

When you're new to a particular pranayama, keep your practice relatively brief, say, 6–12 breaths. This is not so much for safety as to help you establish two habits that are crucial for effective practice: proper breathing mechanics and full concentration at all times.

Once you get into a flow with the technique, practice as long as you can maintain full, relaxed attention to—or better still, absorption in—what you're doing, and as long as it's enjoyable. At some point you'll feel an inner call to set pranayama aside and meditate. Do it.

Add the Power of Your Mind

Just as in asana practice, the more clearly you attune your mind with a specific benefit of a pranayama—relaxation, vitality, calming the nervous system, focusing the mind, upliftment, etc.—the more you'll experience that benefit.

Therefore infuse your practice with whatever you seek: For example, Chandra Bheda Pranayama (Expanding Moon Breath) is a calming technique, so practice it as calmly as you can. Dirgha Pranayama I (Full Yogic Breath) is an invigorating technique, so practice it with calm enthusiasm.

You can do even more with pranayama than with asanas, however, because pranayama quiets the breath and heart, which in turn quiets the mind—and the calmer your mind, the more powerful it is. The mind is most powerful when the breath is still: when you retain the breath internally or especially, externally, without strain. At such times, silent affirmation can be a powerful aid to cultivating any positive quality. Even when the breath moves once again, it can be effective to affirm that positive quality during the inhalation—feel that you're filling yourself with that quality as well as with air—and feel with the exhalation that, along with the air from the lungs, you're expelling any contrary qualities.

For excellent sources of affirmations, see Appendix B: Further Exploration.

Cautions

Because pranayamas move energy, not just air, even the basic ones can have strong effects. Therefore two commonsense cautions are in order:

- Practice with awareness. If you begin to feel agitated, light-headed, nervous, emotional, overheated, or restless, then either it's the wrong technique for you at that particular time, or you're practicing it improperly, or you've practiced it too long. In any case, stop your practice, at least for that session, and simply breathe naturally instead.
- Certain physical conditions, such as cardiovascular disease and pregnancy, call for conservative pranayama practice: retain the breath only for short periods, if at all, and don't overly prolong the inhalations and exhalations. When in doubt, consult your physician.

5.2—BASIC PRANAYAMA TECHNIQUES

A violinist may feel inspiration, but if he doesn't learn techniques that have been developed through the experience of great musicians, he will never become more than an inspired amateur. Yoga techniques, in the same way, are necessary to help you plumb the inner silence.

—PARAMHANSA YOGANANDA

Diaphragmatic Breathing (aka Belly Breathing, Abdominal Breathing)

Diaphragmatic breathing is not so much a pranayama technique as the natural pattern of healthy, relaxed breathing—a pattern that, unfortunately, many people don't follow (often due to stress). Still, for reference purposes it's convenient to give it a specific name.

In fact, *all* breathing involves the diaphragm: it moves down to cause the inhalation and push the belly outward; it relaxes up to cause the exhalation and allow the belly to come back in (see diagram). I append the term "diaphragmatic" to emphasize the value of *feeling* the movements of the diaphragm. Although such feeling is not vital to most of the pranayamas in this book, it's helpful in certain cases.

Technique

Sit or stand upright, or lie supine. Close your eyes, and lift your gaze toward the spiritual eye. Place one hand on your navel, as a learning aid. As you inhale, feel your abdomen pushing into your hand. As you exhale, feel your abdomen relaxing back in. Take several breaths with the hand on the navel, then remove your hand and continue breathing in the same way for a few minutes.

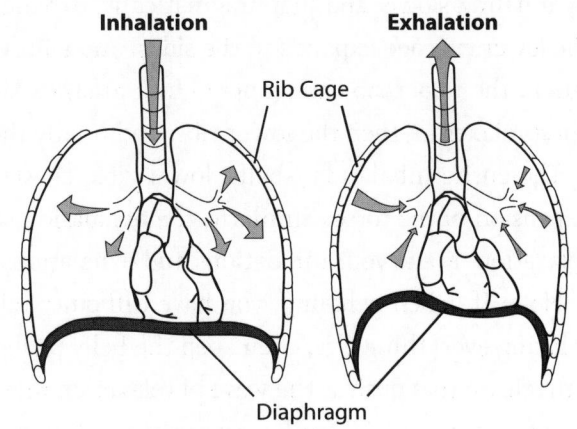

Inhalation Exhalation

Rib Cage

Diaphragm

Your rib cage, too, will expand and contract a bit as you breathe, but focus your attention more on the expansion and relaxation of the abdomen. Make your inhalations and exhalations equal.

Unless otherwise instructed, breathe diaphragmatically in the asanas, pranayamas, meditation, and throughout your day.

Diaphragmatic Breathing becomes a pranayama technique when you begin to lengthen your inhalations and exhalations (keeping them equal), and/or gradually, without strain, lengthen the retentions (most commonly, internal retention).

Dirgha Pranayama I—Full Yogic Breath (aka 3-Part Breathing)

Although the Full Yogic Breath is an energizing practice, it's also calming if you stay within your limits. As your practice deepens, the waves of expansion and relaxation of the torso will seem to be the natural result of the rising and descending energy currents in the spine—as indeed they are, because it's movements of energy that cause the physical body to breathe. The Full Yogic Breath will help you begin to perceive those energy currents more clearly, and learn to work with them more effectively.

Technique

Sit upright, close your eyes, and lift your gaze toward the spiritual eye. Begin a *full* breath by inhaling slowly and diaphragmatically, expanding the belly. As you continue inhaling, the lower rib cage expands to the sides, and a little bit in back. As you complete your inhalation, the upper rib cage (upper chest area) expands. Exhale slowly in reverse order: the chest relaxes in, then the lower ribs, and finally the abdomen.

The entire inhalation—belly, lower ribs, chest—should be a seamless, upward wave of expansion of the torso. Similarly, the exhalation should be a seamless, downward wave of relaxation. Make your inhalations and exhalations equal, and don't strain.

Note: If, when exhaling, you have difficulty relaxing the chest without simultaneously relaxing everything else, then keep the belly pushed out as you begin your exhalation. You can release that push as the wave of relaxation moves down through the torso. This practice is only a learning aid; work toward not needing to exert effort to keep the belly pushed out.

Over time, lengthen your inhalations and exhalations, and add retention (most commonly, internal retention). Lengthen your retentions as you're able. If you like, mentally chant AUM at the spiritual eye while you retain the breath.

Variations

• More advanced: As your practice deepens, concentrate on the energy moving in your astral spine: upward toward the spiritual eye with the upward wave of physical expansion, and downward toward the base of the spine with the downward wave of physical relaxation. Try eventually to make the astral breath your primary experience during this technique. Don't let the eyes turn upward and downward as though following the astral currents; keep your gaze lifted toward the spiritual eye, behind closed eyelids.

• More advanced: Combine the Full Yogic Breath with Ujjayi Pranayama (Victorious Breath), with any of the pranayama techniques practiced with Vishnu Mudra (Symbol of Vishnu), or with bandhas.

Dirgha Pranayama II—Full Yogic Breath Flow

This vitalizing and purifying technique is especially effective for sweeping away moods, self-centeredness, and lethargy, and for cultivating expansiveness and upliftment. Move and breathe slowly and smoothly, feeling that the breath—or better still, prana—is moving your body. Use willpower, concentration, and visualization to sweep energy through your body, aided by the breath and the natural magnetism of your hands.

Technique

From Tadasana, exhale as you relax into a forward bend; finish the exhalation as you reach your lowest point.

Then begin a full yogic inhalation, and feel the breath lifting you, as though inflating your body like a balloon. Glide your hands up the front of the body, not quite touching it, palms facing the body and slightly up, elbows out to the sides. Try to feel the magnetism of the hands lifting energy up through the body.

Complete the inhalation with a graceful overhead stretch of the arms, as though offering the life-force back to its Source. Hold the stretch and the breath for a moment.

With a full yogic exhalation, return to the forward bend position; as you do so, glide the hands down the front of the body, not quite touching it, palms facing the body and slightly down, elbows out to the sides.

Continue for 3–5 more breaths. With each inhalation, feel that you're not only lifting energy

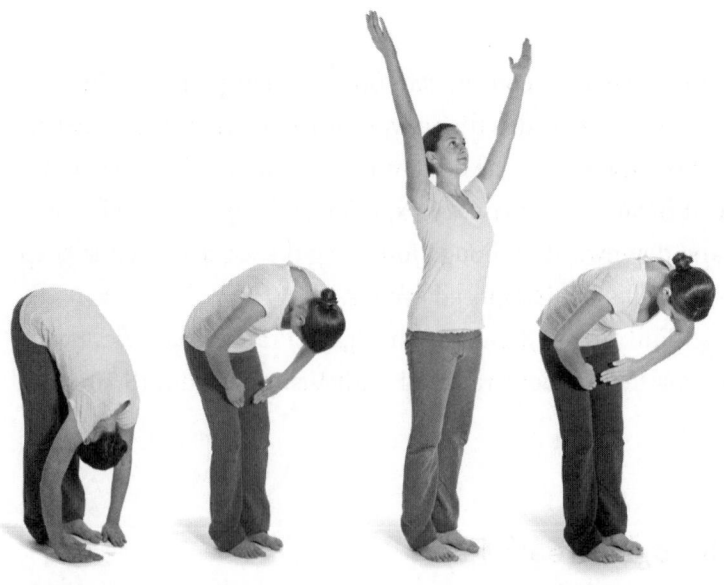

to the brain, but also bringing strength, vitality, and joy into every body cell, from the toes to the crown of your head. With each exhalation, feel that you're wiping away any weakness, fatigue, tension, or negativity. Make your inhalations and exhalations equal.

After your last inhalation and upward-opening stretch, slowly exhale as you circle the hands out to your sides and down. Pause in Tadasana.

Note: If it's more comfortable for your back, keep your knees slightly bent throughout the movements of this technique—especially when practicing without the benefit of prior warm-up exercises. If you have a healthy spine, you can roll up and down, vertebra by vertebra, keeping your knees slightly bent. It's safer for your spine, however, to keep the spine straight for most of this movement, as you do when entering and exiting Padahastasana (Hand-to-the-Foot Pose).

Variation

• Easier: If you find it difficult to combine this sequence of bodily movements with full yogic inhalations and exhalations, then simply breathe diaphragmatically instead.

Double Breathing

When practiced with vigor and deep, strong breaths, Double Breathing brings a double dose of life-force into the body, clarifies the mind, and releases tension from both body and mind. Use it to prepare for vigorous outward activity, to release stress or physical tension, to prime yourself before entering a difficult situation, to prepare for meditation, or anytime you need a pick-me-up. This practice should always be brief; even then, stay within yourself, and stop if you begin to feel light-headed.

Technique

Stand or sit upright. Begin with a two-part inhalation through your nose: a short, sharp inhalation, then a long, strong inhalation. It's a full breath, not a chest breath, so lead the inhalation with expansion of your belly, just as in diaphragmatic breathing. Then exhale through both nose and mouth in two parts: a short, sharp exhalation, followed by a long, strong exhalation—making a breathy, unvocalized sound: "Huh, Huhhhhhh." (Most of the air will naturally go out through the mouth. Don't force it through the nose as well; simply keep the nose relaxed and open.)

Double breaths usually should be quite strong and full. Make your inhalations and exhalations equal. Do 3–6 repetitions.

Variation

• As you double inhale, tense your entire body in a smooth progression, from relaxation to high tension. Retain your breath briefly and vibrate the body with tension. Then, as you double exhale, relax the body in a smooth progression, from high tension to complete relaxation. This variation both energizes the body and helps release tension, including unconsciously-held tension.

Ujjayi Pranayama—Victorious Breath

Ujjayi slows your inhalations and exhalations, and internalizes the mind, helping you enter naturally into meditation. It can also heighten your awareness of the astral breath, thereby helping you gain more control over the spinal energies in general.

Technique

Sit upright, close your eyes, and lift your gaze toward the spiritual eye. Inhale slowly and diaphragmatically through the nose; keep the throat slightly constricted near the epiglottis so that the breath makes a gentle sound. This sound will help you to feel the passage of breath in the throat. It's similar to the sound you make when fogging a mirror—"haaaaaa"—although in Ujjayi your lips remain closed, so the sound is more internal. It might remind you of ocean waves washing ashore, or of a distant waterfall.

Exhale through the nose in the same fashion, with your lips closed and throat slightly constricted. Concentrate on the feeling of the breath moving in and out through the throat. Because the throat is narrowed, the breath will flow more slowly, and thus each breath cycle will last longer. Enjoy that slower pace, and keep your inhalations and exhalations smooth and equal.

Over time, lengthen your inhalations and exhalations, and add retention (most commonly, internal retention). Lengthen your retentions as you're able. If you like, mentally chant AUM at the spiritual eye while you retain the breath.

Variations

• More advanced: As your practice deepens, shift your concentration to the spine near the throat; try to feel the astral breath as it passes that point. Gradually expand that local awareness of the astral breath to awareness of the astral breath throughout its entire course: as you inhale, concentrate on the energy rising from the base of the spine all the way to the spiritual eye; as you exhale, concentrate on energy returning to the base of the spine. Feel as though the sound of Ujjayi is made as much by the movements of the astral breath as by the movements of the physical breath. Don't let the eyes turn upward and downward as though following the astral currents; keep your gaze lifted toward the spiritual eye, behind closed eyelids.
• More advanced: Combine Ujjayi with the Dirgha Pranayama I (Full Yogic Breath), with any of the pranayama techniques done with Vishnu Mudra (Symbol of Vishnu), or with bandhas.

Sitkari Pranayama—Hissing Breath

Sitkari cools the body, soothes the nervous system, and induces physical and mental relaxation. Concentrate on the cooling sensation that arises from this practice, and visualize that sensation spreading throughout the body.

Technique

Sit upright, close your eyes, and lift your gaze toward the spiritual eye. Bring your upper and lower teeth together or nearly together, with your jaw soft and relaxed. Place your tongue gently against the teeth, and inhale smoothly through your mouth with a hissing sound; concentrate on the coolness as the breath enters your mouth. Keep your tongue, mouth, and lips relaxed as you inhale; don't grimace.

Close your lips and retain the breath, enjoying the cool sensation. Then, keeping your lips closed, exhale through your nose and feel the exhalation helping coolness to penetrate up into your brain, and spread throughout your nervous system.

Make your inhalations and exhalations equal; retain the breath as long as you're comfortably enjoying the cooling sensation.

Sitali Pranayama—Cooling Breath

Sitali can be even more effective than Sitkari at cooling the body, soothing the nervous system, and inducing physical and mental relaxation. Concentrate on the cooling sensation—and visualize that cooling sensation spreading through the entire body. To practice Sitali, you must be able to curl your tongue into the shape of a tube; if you're unable to do so, practice Sitkari Pranayama instead.

Technique

Sit upright, close your eyes, and lift your gaze toward the spiritual eye. Place your tongue between your lips (not protruding beyond them) and curl it into a tube. Inhale slowly through that tube, and concentrate on the coolness that you feel at the tip of your tongue and at the back of your throat. Then withdraw your tongue, close your lips, and retain your breath while enjoying that cool sensation. Exhale slowly through your nose, feeling this coolness penetrating up into your brain and spreading throughout your nervous system. Make your inhalations and exhalations equal; retain the breath as long as comfortable.

Your inhalations should be gentle, not forced, so that most of the coolness is felt at the tip of the tongue. The cool sensation at the back of the throat is caused primarily by extending the cool sensation from the tip of the tongue back into the throat, and only secondarily by the rush of air into the throat. The back of the throat is very near the spine, and feeling coolness there will help you distribute that coolness throughout the nervous system.

5.3—PRANAYAMA WITH VISHNU MUDRA

As you inhale, feel that you are drawing strength, courage, and joy up your spine to the brain. While retaining the breath, mentally affirm the positive state of consciousness that you are trying to develop. As you exhale, feel that you are throwing out of your body all opposing states of weakness, discouragement, and sorrow. If you have a specific problem, physical or mental, you may use this technique to affirm the opposite state of well-being, and to throw the negative condition out of your system.

—SWAMI KRIYANANDA

The next three techniques call for breathing through one nostril at a time, with the other nostril lightly held closed. Traditionally, one closes the nostrils using a special hand position called Vishnu Mudra (Symbol of Vishnu[10]) as indicated in the photo captions below.

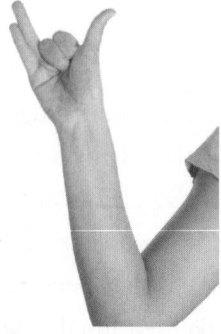
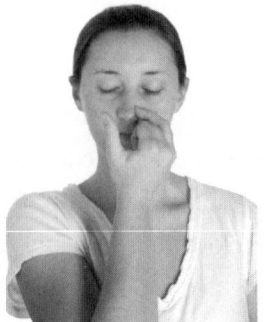
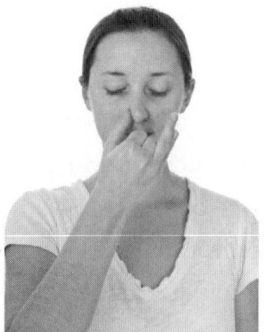
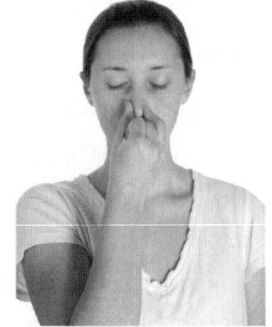

Vishnu Mudra: Hold the tips of the right index and middle fingers against the palm, and extend the thumb and other two fingers

To close the left nostril, press lightly on it with the tips of the little and ring fingers.

To close the right nostril, press lightly on it with the tip of the thumb.

While retaining the breath, press lightly on both nostrils to hold them closed.

---

[10]   To yogis, Vishnu symbolizes the aspect of God that sustains creation.

Practice Tips

- If the traditional mudra is uncomfortable for your hand, you can instead rest the tips of the right index and middle fingers at the point between the eyebrows.
- Breathe fully but not forcefully; the techniques themselves will bring about the indicated results if you stay relaxed and focused.
- Relax your face and breathe with the torso; don't suck air through your one open nostril as though it were a soda straw.
- Since you're breathing only through one nostril at a time, your inhalations and exhalations will be longer than usual; enjoy those longer, slower movements of the breath.

Chandra Bheda Pranayama—Expanding Moon Breath

Chandra Bheda promotes calmness when you feel restless, inwardness when you've been too outward, and relaxation when you're emotionally upset. Choose one of these effects, and as you inhale, feel/visualize that effect growing stronger, fed by the rising energy in the spine. As you exhale, feel/visualize that the expulsion of the breath, aided by the downward current of energy, is helping you to expel any contrary tendencies.

Technique

Sit upright, close your eyes, and lift your gaze toward the spiritual eye. Bring your right hand into Vishnu Mudra, with the thumb next to the right nostril, and the ring and little fingers next to the left nostril.

Close the right nostril with the thumb and inhale through the left nostril. Next, close both nostrils and retain the breath. Then open the right nostril and exhale.

Upon finishing the exhalation, close the right nostril, open the left nostril, and inhale. At first, do just 8–12 breaths total; once you've found the flow of this technique, practice longer.

When first learning this technique, use equal inhalations, exhalations, and retentions. Over time, try to lengthen the inhalations and exhalations, and try to lengthen the retentions even more (without strain).

Variations

- As you retain your breath, chant "AUM" silently and rhythmically at the spiritual eye; feel each repetition of AUM strengthening the desired effect of the practice.

- More advanced: Combine this technique with Dirgha Pranayama I (Full Yogic Breath) or with Ujjayi Pranayama (Victorious Breath).
- More advanced: During internal retention, add Jalandhara Bandha (Chin Lock), which will help you lengthen the retention.

Surya Bheda Pranayama—Expanding Sun Breath

This technique increases your energy when you feel lethargic, your focus when you feel scattered, and your clarity when you feel foggy or confused. Choose one of these effects, and as you inhale, feel/visualize that effect growing stronger, fed by the rising energy in the spine. As you exhale, feel/visualize that the expulsion of the breath, aided by the downward current of energy, is helping you to expel any contrary tendencies.

Technique

Sit upright, close your eyes, and lift your gaze toward the spiritual eye. Bring your right hand into Vishnu Mudra, with the thumb next to the right nostril, and the ring and little fingers next to the left nostril.

Close the left nostril with the ring and little fingers, and inhale through the right nostril. Next, close both nostrils and retain the breath. Then open the left nostril and exhale.

Upon finishing the exhalation, close the left nostril, open the right nostril, and inhale. At first, do just 8–12 breaths total; once you've found the flow of this technique, practice longer.

When first learning this technique, use equal inhalations, exhalations, and retentions. Over time, try to lengthen the inhalations and exhalations, and try to lengthen the retentions even more (without strain).

Variations

- As you retain your breath, chant "AUM" silently and rhythmically at the spiritual eye, feeling each repetition of AUM strengthening the desired effect of the practice.
- More advanced: Combine this technique with Dirgha Pranayama I (Full Yogic Breath) or with Ujjayi Pranayama (Victorious Breath).
- More advanced: During internal retention, add Jalandhara Bandha (Chin Lock), which will help you lengthen the retention.

Nadi Shodhanam—Alternate Nostril Breathing

This pranayama is ideal for promoting mental poise and deeper inner awareness, and especially for balancing and harmonizing the ascending and descending currents of energy in the spine. Feel each inhalation blending into the preceding exhalation, and each exhalation blending with the preceding inhalation—each helping to balance the other and bring you ever closer to breathlessness, and to the perfect stillness beyond the breath.

Technique

Sit upright, close your eyes, and lift your gaze toward the spiritual eye. Bring your right hand into Vishnu Mudra, with the thumb next to the right nostril, and the ring and little fingers next to the left nostril.

Close the right nostril with the thumb and inhale through the left nostril. Next, close both nostrils and retain the breath. Then open the right nostril and exhale.

Upon finishing your exhalation, inhale through the right nostril. Then close both nostrils and retain the breath. Finally, open the left nostril and exhale.

These two complete breaths constitute one cycle of Nadi Shodhanam. At first, do just 6 cycles (12 breaths); once you've found the flow of this technique, practice longer.

When first learning this technique, use equal inhalations, exhalations, and retentions. Over time, try to lengthen the inhalations and exhalations, and try to lengthen the retentions even more (without strain).

Variations

- As you retain your breath, chant "AUM" silently and rhythmically at the spiritual eye, feeling each repetition of AUM strengthening the desired effect of the practice.
- More advanced: Combine this technique with Dirgha Pranayama I (Full Yogic Breath) or with Ujjayi Pranayama (Victorious Breath).
- More advanced: During internal retention, add Jalandhara Bandha (Chin Lock), which will help you lengthen the retention.

5.4—PRANAYAMA WITH BANDHAS

The essence of Yoga is the silence and receptivity that the practice of the techniques induces in the mind.

—PARAMHANSA YOGANANDA

Once you have sound breathing mechanics—they're important, *really*—and have found a natural flow with some of the basic pranayama techniques described above, you'll experience the joy of a quiet, serene breath. You'll begin to feel less stress in daily life. Your mind will be quieter, and your meditations will become deeper and more enjoyable. You might even taste the higher joy of a bit of breathlessness.

Then if you want a deeper inner quiet, the bandhas can help. To engage a bandha, you close or tighten a certain area of the body, thereby concentrating energy in that area, or channeling energy in a particular direction. The goal, as always, is to quiet the breath—and thereby the mind—as well as to bring energy to the brain, or keep it there.

There are three main bandhas in Hatha Yoga. They're quite simple, and they have a variety of applications and variations. We'll explore their highest use: as adjuncts to pranayama practice and to the quest for higher consciousness.

Practice Tips

- It's best to practice bandhas—especially Uddiyana Bandha (Stomach Lift)—on an empty stomach.
- Sit in a comfortable upright position, with your spine straight, eyes closed, and gaze lifted toward the spiritual eye.
- Engage each bandha with calm, sensitive awareness, not sharply or forcefully. Never hold a bandha to the point of strain.
- The physical act of engaging or releasing a bandha can be distracting. Therefore try to lengthen your inhalations, exhalations, and especially your retentions—without strain or getting out of breath—so that those distractions won't happen as often.
- As your breath and mind grow quieter, the physical act of engaging a bandha should become subtler, so as not to disrupt that quiet.

Mula Bandha—Root Lock

Mula Bandha helps you establish and strengthen an overall upward direction of energy in the astral spine. The bandha's upward push from beneath the base of the astral spine creates an upward energetic influence that often will linger even after you release the bandha.

Technique

Focus your concentration on the center of the pelvic floor (the perineum) and, through muscular contraction, draw that area upward. The contraction should be light, without strain. When you release the bandha, be sure to relax the pelvic floor completely.

At first, you may be unable to engage Mula Bandha without also contracting the anal sphincter muscles. With practice, however, you'll become able to keep the anal sphincter muscles relaxed during the bandha.

Note: Anatomy experts do not agree on whether the pelvic floor and perineum are the same, or on how they might differ. For our purposes, fine distinctions are not important, because bandhas are about energy, not physical anatomy. Just think of contracting (lifting upward) the center of the very bottom of the pelvic region—or better still, if you can feel the spinal energy currents, then lift upward from just below the base of the astral spine.

Pranayama with Mula Bandha

Mula Bandha's most natural pranayama companions are Diaphragmatic Breathing, Dirgha Pranayama I (Full Yogic Breath), Ujjayi Pranayama (Victorious Breath), and the three techniques that use Vishnu Mudra.

As you inhale, feel that you're drawing prana up the spine to the brain. Then engage Mula Bandha, and retain the breath as long as comfortable; feel the bandha pushing even more energy to the brain. Then release the bandha and exhale; feel a continuing upward energetic influence in the spine, even as the astral breath descends the spine.

Variation

• More advanced: You can instead (or even also) engage Mula Bandha after an exhalation; retain the breath externally as long as comfortable, then release the bandha and inhale.

Uddiyana Bandha—Stomach Lift

There are strenuous versions of Uddiyana Bandha, but in pranayama practice, apply the bandha gently, and usually with the breath held out. Used sensitively, Uddiyana Bandha can help you cultivate the breathless state. Used insensitively, it will agitate your mind, energy, and body—and make you not want to use the bandha anymore. To get the most out of this technique, align your practice sensitively with the goal: breathlessness.

Technique

As you finish an exhalation, lightly engage your abdominal muscles; smoothly and gently squeeze in toward your spine, and slightly upward. Hold this abdominal lock as long as comfortable, externally retaining the breath. When you need to inhale, relax the abdominal contraction and let your belly expand with the inhalation.

Pranayama with Uddiyana Bandha

Uddiyana Bandha's most natural pranayama companions are Diaphragmatic Breathing, Dirgha Pranayama I (Full Yogic Breath), Ujjayi Pranayama (Victorious Breath), and the three techniques that use Vishnu Mudra.

Variation

• You can instead (or also) apply Uddiyana Bandha *gently* after an inhalation. This variation focuses less on stopping the breath, and more on helping you concentrate energy in the upper astral spine, as you do in Parvatasana (Seated Mountain Pose). As always, retain the breath as long as comfortable.

Jalandhara Bandha—Chin Lock

Jalandhara is an effective mind-quieter, bringing a deeper experience of calmness and expansion of consciousness. Because the gaze may tend to drop as you lower your chin, be sure to keep your eyes turned toward the spiritual eye.

Technique

Gently press your chin to your chest; rest it in the notch between the two collarbones

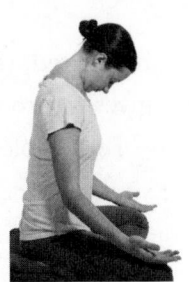

(clavicles). The neck and throat should remain mostly relaxed. Keep the chest lifted, as though rising to meet the chin. Relax your head and face, and lift your gaze toward the spiritual eye.

If your chin does not reach your chest, bring it as close as you can, and tuck it into the neck instead, without strain.

Pranayama with Jalandhara Bandha

Jalandhara's most natural pranayama companions are Diaphragmatic Breathing, Dirgha Pranayama I (Full Yogic Breath), Ujjayi Pranayama (Victorious Breath), and the three techniques that use Vishnu Mudra.

As you inhale, feel that you're drawing prana up the spine to the brain. Then engage Jalandhara Bandha, and retain the breath as long as comfortable; feel the bandha helping to lock energy in the brain, and to focus energy and awareness at the spiritual eye. Then lift your chin to its normal position and exhale; feel much of that energy and awareness remaining at the spiritual eye, even as energy descends the spine with the breath.

Variation

• More advanced: You can instead (or even also) engage Jalandhara Bandha after an exhalation; retain the breath externally as long as comfortable, then release the bandha and inhale.

Combining Bandhas

You can combine two or more bandhas with certain simple pranayama techniques, such as Diaphragmatic Breathing, Dirgha Pranayama I (Full Yogic Breath), and Ujjayi Pranayama (Victorious Breath). These combinations can take you deeper into inner stillness, closer to the breathless state.

Such combinations require an extra measure of coordination and sensitivity, however, else the practice will be merely physical, perhaps even agitating. Remember: if you want to go into a state of deep stillness, you must sensitively harmonize your practice with that state.

As usual, breathe through the nose, use equal inhalations and exhalations, and where instructed, retain the breath as long as comfortable. Practice until the technique naturally gives way to meditation, or until you feel to stop.

Let's explore one such practice, with several variations. Before you try it, be sure that your practice of each separate bandha with pranayama is smooth and easy.

Pranayama with Mula and Jalandhara Bandha

After you inhale, retain the breath, engage Mula Bandha, then engage Jalandhara Bandha. Retain the breath as long as comfortable; concentrate your energy and awareness at the spiritual eye, yet also feel prana still rising toward the brain due to Mula Bandha. As you prepare to exhale, lift the chin to its normal position (thus releasing Jalandhara Bandha); then release Mula Bandha, *and* exhale.

After your final exhalation, sit still and feel prana rising up through the throat to the spiritual eye, separately from the astral breath. Feel your consciousness lifting along with that rising prana.

As you become familiar with this practice, its various components will cease to be separate steps, and will flow together naturally.

Variations

• More advanced: In addition to engaging Mula and Jalandhara with internal retention, engage Uddiyana Bandha with external retention as long as comfortable. Release Uddiyana to begin the next inhalation.

• More advanced (Bahya Pranayama): Engage all three bandhas—Uddiyana, then Mula, then Jalandhara—upon completing the exhalation, and retain the breath externally as long as comfortable. When you need to inhale, release Jalandhara, then Mula, then Uddiyana as you begin your inhalation. Omit the bandhas during internal retention; you can even omit internal retention itself.

5.5—VIGOROUS PRANAYAMA

Many students of Yoga make the mistake of thinking that by their will power alone, exerted through the daily practice of breathing exercises, physical postures, and meditation techniques, they will attain cosmic consciousness. Their approach to the spiritual life is almost as if God were a sort of divine mountain, to be conquered in a spirit of mountaineering bravado! That is hardly the spirit in which to approach Yoga, that highest of spiritual sciences!

—SWAMI KRIYANANDA

Now for two techniques that can be extraordinarily powerful aids to a quieter, more focused, more uplifted mind, and to a deeper meditation. Practiced incorrectly or in excess, however, they can agitate the mind or emotions—or worse, and more dangerous, they can force more energy through your body than its "energy circuitry" can handle. Therefore be sure to follow these additional guidelines:

Practice Tips

- Practice these techniques only if you have good breathing mechanics, prior experience with pranayamas, good powers of self-observation and self-honesty, and the common sense to stop if you feel any discomfort, dizziness, or agitation.
- Begin with a brief practice, and slowly build to a longer practice.
- Although the abdominal muscles and diaphragm work hard in these techniques, the rest of your body should move as little as possible. Be especially sure to keep your shoulders still and your face relaxed.
- Maintain a steady, even rhythm of breathing; an irregular rhythm will agitate you. If you lose the rhythm, stop and take a few easy diaphragmatic breaths before resuming the practice.
- Incorrect or excessive practice can lead to hyperventilation. Although some people like that light-headed "high," by no means is it higher consciousness. These techniques should make you feel clear-minded and focused, not spaced out.
- Although similar, these two techniques can have quite different effects. It's usually best not to practice both within the same routine.

Kapalabhati Pranayama—Breath of Fire (aka Skull-Shining Breath)

Kapalabhati lifts your energy and awareness to the spiritual eye, and brings to the mind a feeling of deep stillness and clarity. It's excellent before meditation.

Technique

Preparation: Sit upright and take several deep, diaphragmatic breaths through the nose. Finish your last exhalation by smoothly yet firmly squeezing the abdomen in, forcing the air out through the nostrils.

Now begin the technique proper: Quickly relax your abdominal muscles so that the abdomen expands forward naturally, and an inhalation flows in through the nose. Then quickly and smoothly squeeze the abdomen inward, causing an exhalation through the nose. All effort should be on the exhalation. Don't *push* your abdomen out; rather, *relax* it out and let the air flow in on its own. Your inhalations and exhalations should be of equal duration.

Continue in this way—relax out to inhale, squeeze in to exhale—doing about one complete breath per second. Keep the shoulders and face relaxed and still; allow only the abdomen to move. Do 12 breaths in all, finishing with one last abdominal squeeze. Then let the body breathe as it will, for at least 5 breaths. After that, you can do another round of 12 breaths. Continue in this way for 3–6 rounds total.

As you gain experience, increase beyond 12 breaths per round and/or beyond 3–6 rounds. Always keep a smooth, even rhythm, and emphasize depth of practice over duration.

Variation

• More advanced: Once you've become comfortable with Kapalabhati, follow your final abdominal contraction with a smooth, slow, full yogic inhalation; focus on lifting energy upward to the spiritual eye as you inhale. Concentrate at the spiritual eye as you retain the breath as long as comfortable, then release the breath with a full yogic exhalation. Practice this up to 3 times, then let go of the breath and simply enjoy the deep inner stillness and clarity.

Bhastrika Pranayama—Bellows Breath

Bhastrika lifts your energy and awareness to the spiritual eye, cleanses the mind of restlessness, and brings a sense of vibrant alertness. It's excellent before meditation. Bhastrika requires even more coordination than Kapalabhati, so practice it sensitively.

Technique

Preparation: Sit upright and take several deep, diaphragmatic breaths through the nose. Finish your last exhalation by smoothly yet firmly squeezing the abdomen in, forcing the air out through the nostrils.

Now begin the technique proper: Quickly push the abdomen back out, thereby causing an inhalation through the nose. Then quickly and smoothly squeeze the abdomen inward, causing an exhalation through the nose. Both movements should be smooth and firm. Your inhalations and exhalations should be of equal duration.

Continue in this way—push out to inhale, squeeze in to exhale—doing about one complete breath per second. Keep the shoulders and face relaxed and still; allow only the abdomen to move. Do 12 breaths in all; finish with one last abdominal squeeze. Then let the body breathe as it will, for at least 5 breaths. After that, you can do another round of 12 breaths. Continue in this way for 3–6 rounds total.

As you gain experience, increase beyond 12 breaths per round and/or beyond 3–6 rounds. Always keep a smooth, even rhythm, and emphasize depth of practice over duration.

Note: It's actually the downward movement of the diaphragm that causes the abdomen to be thrust out. If you've developed a conscious awareness of the diaphragm's movements in such basic techniques as Diaphragmatic Breathing and Dirgha Pranayama I (Full Yogic Breath), it will serve you well in Bhastrika.

Variation

• More advanced: Once you've become comfortable with Bhastrika, follow your final abdominal contraction with a smooth, slow, full yogic inhalation; focus on lifting energy upward to the spiritual eye as you inhale. Concentrate at the spiritual eye as you retain the breath as long as comfortable, then release the breath with a full yogic exhalation. Practice this up to 3 times, then let go of the breath and simply enjoy the vibrant inner stillness and alertness.

Chapter
SIX

Meditation

The higher teachings of Yoga take one beyond techniques, and show the Yoga practitioner how to direct his concentration in such a way as not only to harmonize human with divine consciousness, but to merge his consciousness in the Infinite.

—PARAMHANSA YOGANANDA

What Is True Meditation?

One hears the word "meditation" so frequently now that its meaning has become blurred. Its aim is not merely to calm your emotions, clear your mind, or relieve stress, although it will do all that. And although true meditation will take you beyond thought, blanking out is not the way to get there. Nor does meditation mean "thinking things over."

In fact, strictly speaking, meditation is not even something one *does*; it's a state of consciousness—a profoundly serene, often joyful, state in which you're beyond thought and beyond perceiving yourself as separate from the rest of creation. There's a vibrant sense of being complete in yourself—and of knowing for certain that "yourself" is much, much more than you had ever imagined. You're experiencing, at long last, something of your own divine essence.

In common usage, however, "meditation" also refers to techniques that can help you reach that state of consciousness. Although absent from most approaches to Hatha Yoga, meditation is integral to Ananda Yoga®, and it's the central practice of the greater spiritual science of Raja Yoga. Only meditation, of all Yoga's many techniques, can take you to Self-realization.

Asanas and pranayamas, however, are excellent adjuncts to meditation. They can do much more than merely prepare your body to sit comfortably; they can calm and internalize your mind, and help you direct your energy and consciousness inward and upward. Then, just as the first stage of a rocket drops away and the second stage takes over to boost a satellite into orbit, so also can meditation techniques lift you toward the lofty state of meditation.

The Yoga tradition offers a variety of meditation techniques, each with its own distinct approach. Ananda Yoga includes three such techniques; here we'll explore the art and science of one of them: the simple yet powerful Hong-Sau technique.[11]

6.1—THE SCIENCE: CONCENTRATE AND CALM THE MIND

Have you ever noticed, when you're deeply engrossed in reading a book, that your breathing has become very shallow or infrequent—or both? This happens whenever you're deeply concentrated: the act of concentrating brings a degree of stillness to your mind, which in turn quiets your breath (i.e., slows it down and/or makes it shallower). You also experience this breath-mind connection when you perform a delicate task such as threading a needle: you need to concentrate, so you instinctively hold your breath, because you know on deeper-than-conscious levels that the breath is an obstacle to concentration.

The breath-mind connection is hardwired into human beings, and the Hong-Sau technique takes advantage of it. You begin by concentrating on the breath. The act of concentrating calms your mind a bit; a calmer mind results in quieter breath. With the breath quieter, you can concentrate more deeply, which calms the mind even more, which in turn makes the breath grow even quieter. Your initial act of concentration has helped you enter a positive feedback loop (see diagram) that will bring you ever-deeper

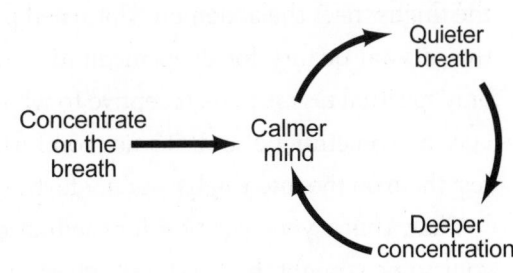

calmness of breath and mind. In Hong-Sau practice, you simply continue in that positive loop; practiced deeply, Hong-Sau can take you all the way to the breathless state. That's the general idea of the Hong-Sau technique. Now let's explore the specifics.

---

[11] The other two techniques require additional preparation. The most advanced of the three is the renowned Kriya Yoga technique. For more information, see Appendix B: Further Exploration.

Preparation

Find a Comfortable Sitting Position

Any comfortable sitting position will do, provided it enables you to keep your spine straight and your body relaxed. The sitting asanas (see Section 4.7) are good positions for meditation; Sukhasana (Easy Pose) and Swastikasana (Auspicious Pose) are easiest for most people, although Sukhasana is not ideal for more than a few minutes. If your spine rounds and/or you feel knee or ankle discomfort in these asanas, and if sitting on a cushion doesn't correct the situation, then sit on a meditation bench or chair (see photos). Whatever position you choose, your knees should be a bit lower than your hip joints, so that you can more easily sit with a straight spine; sit on a cushion, if necessary, to ensure that.

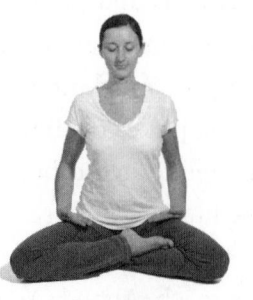
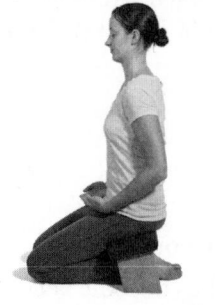
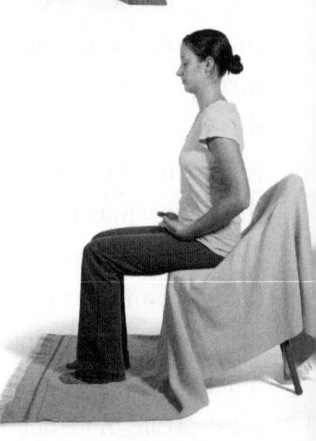

If you sit on a chair, place your feet flat on the floor (or on a cushion), and sit away from the back of the chair. If the chair seat slopes downward, front to back, then sit on the front edge of the seat, else the slope will make it difficult to keep your spine straight. If the front edge of the seat presses uncomfortably on the backs of your legs, place a cushion under your feet to raise your knees, making sure your knees remain a bit lower than your hips.

Next, rest your hands, palms facing upward, on the thighs where the thighs meet the abdomen. Upturned palms help you be receptive, a vital quality for deep meditation; after all, your one and only spiritual task is to be receptive to what you already are, not to become something else. If it's not comfortable to have your hands close to your body, then rest them on the mid-thighs, but not farther away that that, lest your shoulders tend to round.

Okay, this is your position for meditation. Stay this way throughout your practice, with your spine straight, body relaxed, chest open, shoulders comfortably back, and belly soft.

Lift Your Gaze Toward the Spiritual Eye

Close your eyes and turn your gaze toward the spiritual eye. Don't try to *see* something; simply keep your eyes relaxed up into this position throughout your meditation.

Instead of closing your eyes, you can keep your eyelids half-open, provided they don't distract you by fluttering. Usually the mind must be quite still in order for the eyelids to be half-open without fluttering.

Relax Body and Mind

Ideally, you've already practiced some Hatha Yoga and are feeling relaxed and revitalized, both physically and mentally. If not, however, do the following two exercises to relax the body, then the mind:

1. *Tense & relax:* Inhale, tense the whole body as you briefly retain the breath, then throw the breath out and relax the entire body. (Use a Double Breath if you like.) Repeat 3–6 times.

2. *Even-Count Breathing (aka Measured Breathing):* Inhale slowly and diaphragmatically through the nose; retain the breath for the same count; exhale through the nose for the same count. Then immediately inhale again, and continue. Increase the count if you like, keeping all three phases of the breath equal and free of strain. Practice this technique for 3–6 breaths.

Body and mind should now be relaxed, ready to meditate.

The Hong-Sau Technique

From now on, breathe only through your nose. Inhale fully, then exhale completely and let go of the breath, no longer controlling it in any way. Practice the following:

- *Watch the breath.*—Focus your attention on the breath wherever you feel it most easily: ideally somewhere in the nose, the higher the better. Don't control, analyze, or mentally comment on the breath; just witness it, feel it, and let the body breathe as it will. If your point of attention shifts higher in the nose during your practice, all the better.

- *Mentally repeat the mantra[12].*—As each breath flows in of its own accord, accompany it silently with the sound "Hong." Don't move your lips or tongue, or tense the throat; just *think* the sound. When the breath flows out of its own accord, accompany it mentally with the sound "Sau" (pronounced "saw"). Hong-Sau is a mantric form of a Sanskrit sentence that means "I am Spirit"; thus, on one level, Hong-Sau is an affirmation. Focus, however, on the naturally flowing breath and on the mental sounds, not on the meaning of the mantra.

---

[12] A *mantra* is a word-formula, the very sound of which (whether repeated outwardly or only inwardly) has a beneficial, transformative effect on one's consciousness.

- *Move the right forefinger.*—As each breath flows in, slightly curl your right forefinger toward the palm. As your breath flows out, relax the forefinger away from the palm. Make the movement small enough that it's not a distraction; its purpose is simply to help you to concentrate on the breath, and to distinguish between inhalation and exhalation when the breath becomes very shallow.

As you continue with the practice, the breath may slow down or become quite shallow; either is a sign of correct practice. If at any time your breathing stops of its own accord, that's even better. Don't force the pause to be longer—remember: you're not controlling the breath—but neither should you hasten the breath to flow again. Just wait, and when the breath flows again of its own accord, resume the technique.

Hong-Sau can bring you into a very still state, beyond the usual distracting chatter of the mind, even to breathlessness. There you'll usually experience, not emptiness, but vibrant awareness of a deep, rejuvenating peace—a peace that is your very essence. Although peace is the most typical result of Hong-Sau practice, you might instead experience another divine quality, such as joy, love, or wisdom. Experiencing any of these qualities is a sign of correct practice. However, don't be discouraged if none of this happens right away; it will come in its own time.

Those are the mechanics of the Hong-Sau technique. Practice it for the first two-thirds to three-quarters of your meditation time; then for the rest of your meditation time:

Go Beyond Technique

Sit quietly, with the same posture of body and eyes. Forget about the mantra, the breath, and the right forefinger. Try to absorb yourself in the inner stillness—or peace, joy, love, or another divine quality if you feel one. Try to *relax upward* into that quality, to *become* that quality. The technique has acted as the second stage of a rocket to lift you to where you can access this higher state, but no technique can take that last step for you; that's the art of meditation (see Section 6.2).

Stay in this state as long as your attentiveness, enjoyment, and time permit. This will strengthen your faculty of intuition and, as Paramhansa Yogananda put it, "you will find yourself in touch with the unexplored reservoir of divine power."

If your mind becomes restless and clamors for something to do—that happens to everyone at times—refocus it by resuming Hong-Sau practice, or by engaging the mind in affirmation, visualization, silent chanting, a mantra, or prayer. Or simply call to the Inner Presence with deep longing, "Reveal Thyself"; then try to feel the divine response in your heart.

Transition into Activity

When it's time to be up and about again, hold onto the feeling of peace (or joy, or love) as long as possible. It will help if you move calmly and gracefully, and try to infuse your daily activities with that peace (or joy, or love). Renew that consciousness regularly by taking short meditation breaks as often as possible, even if only for a breath or two.

Practical Meditation Tips

- *Emphasize quality over quantity.*—Meditate at least once every day; twice a day is even better. Long meditations are good, but depth of meditation is far more important than duration. It's better to meditate deeply for 5 minutes than to daydream or drowse for 30 minutes. Daydreaming and sleeping are *not* meditation; they are, in fact, two of the most insidious, hard-to-break habits that can plague your efforts to meditate. Don't *ever* let either of them gain a foothold in your practice. Once a week, make time for a longer practice; a longer, *deeper* meditation will help you break new ground in your meditative life.

- *Find your ideal times.*—You can meditate anytime, but the best time for meditation is usually right after your practice of asana and pranayama. Sunrise, noon, sunset, and midnight are said to be especially good times for meditation; the energy flow in your body is more balanced during these "rest points" in nature. In any case, meditate at the same time(s) every day; regularity will help you feel like meditating at those times. Although it's fine to practice Hong-Sau right after a meal, your experience will usually be better if you meditate when your stomach is empty.

- *Create a sacred space.*—In your home, set aside a meditation-only space: a separate room, or a screened-off portion of your bedroom. Make an altar, and adorn it with items that inspire you: pictures of saints, divine images, flowers, crystals, or other special objects from nature. Your space will soon develop a peaceful, uplifting vibration that will help you meditate more deeply.

- *Face east or north.*—Yoga teaches that it's ideal to face east when you meditate, for then you'll receive an assist from certain subtle, uplifting currents of consciousness that come from that direction. If you cannot face east, then try to face north. East is said to be the direction of enlightenment, and north the direction of liberation (divine union).

- *Insulate yourself.*—Sit on a woolen blanket when meditating, for wool helps insulate your energy from the downward pull of subtle gravity. A silk cloth on top of the woolen blanket will provide even more insulation. If you sit on a chair, the blanket should run over the back of the chair, over the seat, and under your feet.

- *Be regular.*—Regular meditation is a key to a fruitful practice and a happier, more productive life. There will be times when your mind tells you, "I don't have time to meditate." Don't believe it. Maybe you can't meditate as long as usual, but do at least a little bit. When you commit to a regular practice—even just 5 minutes a day—and follow through on your commitment, the Universe will find ways to support your practice.

6.2—THE ART: ATTUNE YOUR MIND TO WHAT YOU SEEK

Just as with asanas and pranayamas, you'll meditate better if you call upon your "artistic" faculties as described in Chapter 1: willpower, concentration, feeling, visualization, positive attitude, and devotion. Above all, open yourself to divine grace; remember, God wants you to meditate deeply enough to feel the divine connection. Here are some aids to practicing the art of Hong-Sau meditation:

Stay Relaxed and Receptive

When you sit to meditate, relax not only your body, but also your mind. The mind is accustomed to making things happen; once armed with a technique, it can all too easily slip into trying to make the state of meditation happen. Well, you can't *make* it happen, and if you try, you'll create tension, which defeats your purpose. You can, however, *receive* the state of meditation. If you practice with relaxed, alert focus, strong aspiration, and a receptive attitude (the upturned palms and open chest will help you be receptive), then meditation—both the practice and the state—will come much more easily and naturally.

Be the Observer

As you watch the breath, cultivate a sense of being apart from it. Instead of feeling, "I am breathing," feel simply that breathing is happening, and you're witnessing it—with your complete attention, but nevertheless, just witnessing.

Cultivate Intensity of Concentration

The longer you stay fully focused on the breath and mantra, the deeper you'll go into that positive feedback loop that I described earlier, and a doorway will open to higher consciousness. Your concentration, however, must be relaxed, calm, and willing; never strain, because tension will keep that doorway closed. You'll stay more relaxed if you choose to be intently interested in the breath, for when you're truly interested in something, concentration becomes natural and effortless.

Find the Flow

Hong-Sau practice might at first seem complicated: upright posture, uplifted gaze, watching the breath, repeating the mantra, moving the right forefinger. But just as with any other multifaceted activity—such as driving a car, using a computer, or cooking—you'll soon get into a natural flow in which the various components blend seamlessly into an enjoyable whole. Try to feel that flow early in your practice; then, like a kayaker paddling with the current, actively cooperate with that flow.

Don't Fight Against Thoughts

Yes, thoughts will arise during your practice, but fighting against them will only make them more prominent and persistent. Instead, accept that they're part of the process, and ignore them. Whenever you catch yourself thinking, simply turn your attention firmly back to the breath and the mantra, as if saying to the thought, "I'll catch up with you later, but right now I'm busy." That's part of the process of meditation: the mind wanders, you bring it back, it wanders again, you bring it back again. As you persevere over time, not yielding to the temptation to continue wandering, you'll retrain your mind to wander less and less.

Enjoy the Pauses

In normal breathing, there's a natural pause after you inhale but before you exhale, and a similar pause after you exhale but before you inhale. Those pauses are precious; as I mentioned in Chapter 5, the mind is quieter and more powerful when the breath isn't flowing. Hong-Sau practice helps to prolong those pauses—naturally—and hence to deepen your inner quiet. Calmly enjoy those pauses, without forcibly lengthening them. Immerse yourself in the inner stillness of the pauses, and feel that stillness continuing in the background even when the breath flows once again. Enjoy your freedom from the breath's constant tendency to agitate your mind and draw your awareness outward.

Meet Higher Consciousness Halfway

If you want to experience divine peace, meditate with the *feeling* of peace. Simply decide to be peaceful, and practice with the relaxed anticipation of more peace to come. Doing so puts you on the wavelength of divine peace; only when you're on that wavelength can you experience divine peace deeply. The same can be said for experiencing any other divine quality, although as noted earlier, Hong-Sau practice most typically leads one to the experience of peace.

Stay Connected

Make the most of the final portion of your meditation time, when you're no longer watching the breath and repeating the mantra, no longer "doing" in any way. It's easy for the mind to wander at this time. To maintain focus, use your intuitive faculty to feel whatever divine quality—peace, joy, calmness, love—remains in the wake of your active practice. Your relaxed willpower and devotion will help keep your attention focused on it. Then offer yourself into that quality, try to *merge* into the divine ocean of that quality. If thoughts come, view them like tiny bubbles floating on the surface; your reality is the vast, eternal ocean, not those insignificant, evanescent bubbles.

Partner with Spirit

Bring the Divine into your meditations. Try to feel the Inner Presence subtly guiding your practice, and gently calling your mind back whenever it wanders. Meditate *with* God, not *for* God. And when you finish your active practice of watching the breath, repeating the mantra, etc., relax upward into an ever-more-intimate connection with your Divine Friend.

———————

There's much more to meditation than this brief introduction, but this is enough to get you well on your way to a deeply rewarding practice. When you're ready for more, see Appendix B: Further Exploration.

Chapter
SEVEN

Yoga as a Way of Life

You will attain superconsciousness more quickly, and not only in meditation, if you seek to attune yourself with it in your daily activities. The more you seek to be guided by intuition, which is an aspect of superconsciousness, the greater success you will meet in every undertaking.

—SWAMI KRIYANANDA

Yoga techniques are valuable tools for spiritual growth, yet we spend most of our waking hours doing other things. If those activities don't support our spiritual practices—or worse, if they work against our efforts—then we won't get very far. That's why lifestyle is such an important part of traditional Yoga.

Yoga takes it beyond lifestyle, too, for it's not only *what* we do that aids or impedes our growth; it's *how* we do it: attitude is supremely important. I touched upon this often in earlier chapters, when emphasizing the value of attuning yourself to the positive attitudes induced by the techniques, and the attitude of partnership with Spirit in all that you do. To gain a deeper understanding of the role of attitude for the yogi, I highly recommend exploring the Bhagavad Gita (see Appendix B: Further Exploration).

In this chapter, I'll focus on a number of areas in which lifestyle tweaks can support your spiritual aspirations. View this as a menu of many options: ways to increase, free, or uplift your energy; to stop wasting energy; or to overcome influences—internal or external—that work against your spiritual growth. Whichever of these ideas you feel inspired to try, make your exploration into an adventure, an experiment, something that's fun to try.

And remember: when you make the effort to rise—whether through techniques, attitude, divine connection, or lifestyle—you generate a magnetism that attracts aid from the Universe. As Paramhansa Yogananda said, "If you resolve firmly to 'try and try again,' God Himself and His angels will come to your aid."

7.1—FIND BALANCE

Yoga teaches—and it's easy to recognize in your own life—that lifestyle extremes will take you out of your center, create tension, deplete your energy, and work against your efforts to grow. It's far wiser to take the middle road of intelligent, commonsense balance. This doesn't mean self-deprivation; it simply means recognizing what takes you where you want to go, and what doesn't—and living accordingly. It's an investment in clarity of mind, mental and spiritual vitality, personal freedom, and above all, happiness.

Unfortunately, we humans find countless ways to be *out* of balance. Here are a few: workaholism, incessant outward activity, addiction to digital devices ("Who, me?"), habitual laziness or procrastination, compulsive physical workouts, sleeping too much or too little, substance abuse (nicotine, drugs, alcohol, even coffee and sugar), too-rigid dietary habits, overeating, lack of personal boundaries, talking too much, constant socializing, isolating yourself from people, too much or too little sexual activity.[13] And let's not forget the greatest imbalance of all: too much emphasis on "I, me, my, and mine."

Apply It to Your Life

Choose one area in which you're ultra-strict with yourself, or ultra-indulgent or lazy, or simply out of balance. (If you can't think of one, hurray for you! But just to be sure, you might ask a friend for an honest opinion.) Then pull back from that extreme—far enough to feel a difference, but not so far that your mind rebels. It's okay if your mind whines a bit, though; just reassure it that this is merely an experiment, and if the experiment hasn't led to greater happiness in, say, 2–4 weeks, you'll cheerfully resume your familiar ways. On the other hand, if by that time you're enjoying newfound balance, your mind will happily support the

---

[13] Yoga warns that overindulgence in sex drains your natural vitality, whereas at the other extreme, unrealistic sexual self-deprivation can lead to tensions and negative psychological repercussions. Each individual needs to find, with complete self-honesty, his or her own middle road.

lifestyle change. Then repeat the experiment in another area in which you've been out of balance. It's an effective way to free up and direct energy in more-productive ways, whether for outward projects or for inner growth.

7.2—CREATE A SUPPORTIVE ENVIRONMENT

Your state of mind is strongly influenced by your environment: the people you're with, the places where you spend time (home, work, leisure), the art and colors around you (including your clothing), the music you listen to, the books you read, the movies you watch, the websites you visit. Make no mistake: everything affects your consciousness. As Paramhansa Yogananda often said, "Environment is stronger than will."

Therefore it's important to find or create spiritually supportive environments, and avoid those that inhibit your growth. Seek out people who are happy, optimistic, generous, serviceful, supportive, positive, and especially, spiritually inclined. Spend time in such high-vibration places as churches and temples, nature, gardens, places of beauty—anywhere that uplifts your energy. On the other hand, try to avoid gossipers, complainers, and people who are restless, negative, greedy, or "energy sponges." Don't frequent bars, casinos, drug- or alcohol-saturated parties, messy places, loud or agitated environments, or anywhere that the overall level of energy or consciousness is low.

The choices aren't always easy—when you realize, for example, that some of your friends are influencing you in directions you don't want to go. But they *are* choices, and there's *always* something you can do to uplift your environment.

Apply It to Your Life

Begin by cultivating greater awareness of the effects that your environments have on you. For each one, ask, "Does this support my aspirations, or not?" Find the answer, in part by analyzing the external environment, but especially by feeling your inner *response* to that environment: Do you feel relaxed, clear-minded, expansive, positive, or uplifted? Or do you feel somewhat nervous, vulnerable, agitated, depressed, or eager to get away? Those inner feelings can be more telling than the outward reality of the place.

Here are a few environment-based ways to support your spiritual aspirations:

- Everyone has positive qualities, even people who don't readily exhibit them. Try to be more aware of positive qualities in the people around you; actively appreciate those qualities—at least with generous thoughts, and sometimes with spoken words. Cultivate the habit of, when you first see someone, bringing one of his or her positive qualities to mind. This will help shield you from negative influences that the person may project—as well as from any that might otherwise come up in you, in response to those influences. It will also be a lot more fun to spend time with that person.

- Spend more time in nature. It's good to *be* in nature, and even better to *immerse* yourself in its vibrations of balance and harmony. Try to feel its slow, natural rhythms, and to feel a part of yourself resonating with those rhythms. As you harmonize with nature, you'll harmonize with your natural Self. To become even more receptive to nature's blessings, consciously appreciate nature, and express your gratitude to it.

- Is your living or working environment pulling you down, yet you can't leave it? Take heart! There is always *something*—and usually, many things—you can do to counter its effects. If it's messy, help to clean it up. If people are negative, find ways to support them without supporting their negativity. If people are fearful, give them extra kindness. Even if there's nothing you can do outwardly to change the situation, you can always work on your *inner* environment: if you feel judgmental, resistant, or resentful about your outer environment, then you're creating a negative inner environment. Upgrade it by refusing to be negative. Instead find something—anything—in your environment that you can be positive about, and cling to that positivity. You'll be much happier, and you might find that your inner upgrade mysteriously upgrades your outer environment as well.

- In your life, is there a shortage of happy, optimistic, generous, serviceful, supportive, positive, and/or spiritually inclined people? They're everywhere; you just might need to look around a bit more, to spend time with new groups of people, to try new activities. And in the meantime, you can always read books or watch movies about the lives of such inspiring people as saints, great leaders, and famous humanitarians.

- God is always with you, in any environment. Remind yourself of the Divine Mother's presence by silently, continuously practicing *japa* (repeating a name of Spirit, or a mantra), or a simple prayer such as "Be with me now. Be with me always." Another approach is to carry on a continuous inner conversation with your Divine Friend. The more your inner environment is filled with His or Her loving, supportive presence—even if, at first, it feels as though you're just pretending—the more your experience of life will improve. For resources that will instruct and inspire you in this direction, see "Cultivating Your Divine Connection" in Appendix B: Further Exploration.

7.3—FIND FREEDOM IN SERVICE

You've felt it: the more you escape the confines of "I, me, my, mine," the happier you are. One excellent way to get out of yourself is to expand your consciousness through the practices of Yoga. Another way is to serve others, support the welfare of others. This doesn't mean that you ignore your own needs; it's just that when you see your own needs in a broader perspective, they seem less pressing, and your difficulties seem less difficult. Serving others takes the focus off "me," thereby relieving a lot of tension, and at the same time correcting misdirected energy.

If you take the attitude of service a step further, and try to serve with conscious awareness of divine energy flowing through you, that awareness can wash away all thought of the small self, and in the process give you a glowing sense of freedom, divine connection, and unlimited possibilities.

Apply It to Your Life

When you think of service, do you think of such major projects as volunteering in another country, or working in a soup kitchen one day each week? Such service is admirable and can be life changing, but there are many smaller, more immediate ways to serve, wherever you are. Each day look for some way—even a very small way—in which you can serve another person: offer to help in some way; run an errand for someone; do an anonymous good deed; give encouragement, a gift, or a compliment; share laughter; smile for no reason. Don't make a big deal of it. Just do it, and enjoy the freedom that it brings. The cost is small, and the payoff can be great, especially if you do it regularly.

In fact, take it a step further: view service, not as occasional favors, but as part of the overall flow of your life. For example, if you have a job, view your duties as service to others rather than merely a means to a paycheck. Be specific: exactly whom are you serving, and in what ways? Infuse your efforts with a sense of caring about those people, and try to feel you're blessing them. If you're an at-home parent, view your daily chores as loving service to your family, and through your family, to everyone they meet. Anytime you think "service" rather than "work," your tasks become easier and you loosen the bonds of ego-consciousness, so that your awareness can soar. You have a lot more fun, too.

7.4—OUTER FITNESS FEEDS INNER FITNESS

Regular healthy exercise is important, not only for physical and psychological health, but also for spiritual health. As Paramhansa Yogananda once urged Swami Kriyananda, "Keep exercised and body fit for God-realization." Don't become obsessed with exercise; just give the body the exercise it needs in order to stay healthy and do what you need it to do.

What is healthy exercise? Put simply, it's a regular regime that brings strength, flexibility, cardiovascular fitness, and vitality. A well-rounded asana practice—even if practiced only on a physical level—will give you strength and flexibility. And if you practice as described in this book, your level of vitality will increase too.[14] Aerobic exercise, in which the heart rate is elevated for a prolonged period, completes the picture by conditioning your cardio-vascular system. Add to the mix a cheerful, positive mental outlook, and you'll have even more vitality.

Apply It to Your Life

In addition to your asana and pranayama practice—you're already doing it, right?—walk vigorously for 20 minutes, 4–5 times each week. In your everyday flow, take advantage of opportunities to walk, even when it's only a short distance. If walking isn't right for you, try swimming, bicycling, cardio equipment at the gym, aerobics classes, anything that safely increases your heart rate. And to make your cardio regime more enjoyable, use that time to work on developing a habitually cheerful, positive mental outlook. On some days this can be more challenging than the cardio workout, but it's well worth the effort.

Don't take any form of physical exercise to extremes—remember balance—but do have a regular exercise program. (It's good to take a positive mental outlook to extremes, however, provided you stay grounded.) Consult your healthcare advisor to develop a program that's appropriate for you.

---

[14] If you want vitality, I highly recommend supplementing your asana practice with the Energization Exercises of Paramhansa Yogananda (see Appendix B: Further Exploration). In addition to deepening your spiritual efforts by teaching you greater awareness of, and control over, the life-force, Energization builds strength, tones the muscles, improves circulation, and increases your overall vitality.

7.5—DIETARY CHOICES CAN HELP

Today it's well known that dietary choices impact physical health. (Many people don't make *wise* dietary choices, but that's another matter.) It's less well known that dietary choices also impact spiritual health. Poor diet will clog the bodily system, drain its energy, and weaken one's practice of asana, pranayama, and meditation. Poor diet can also drag down one's overall state of awareness: the body is forced to spend too much energy dealing with what's being put into it, energy that *could* have been lifted to the brain to raise awareness.

Paramhansa Yogananda strongly encouraged a vegetarian diet, and wrote extensively on dietary matters. He also warned against becoming a food fanatic (remember balance); he advocated instead a commonsense approach that he called "proper eatarianism": find a dietary regime that supports your good health and vitality, and stick to it. Here are a few of his simple guidelines for finding your own proper-eatarian diet (for more information, see Appendix B: Further Exploration):

- Eat foods that have a calming, harmonizing effect on your system: fresh fruits, nuts, raw or lightly cooked vegetables, whole grains, and fresh dairy products.
- Avoid foods that irritate, excite, weaken, or clog your system: excessively spicy food, alcoholic beverages, too many carbohydrates, stimulants (yes, that includes too much caffeine), junk food, overly processed food, iced drinks, frozen foods, and stale or devitalized food.
- Abstain as much as possible from beef, pork, poultry, and fish. They can clog your digestive system, and agitate or dull your state of mind. At the very least, avoid beef and pork, and eat poultry and fish less frequently. Nourishing vegetable forms of protein are easily available.
- Were Yogananda to speak today, I'm confident that he would recommend eating only organically grown foods. In his lifetime, pesticides, herbicides, chemical additives, preservatives, genetic engineering, growth hormones, antibiotics for animals, etc., were not the big issues that they are today, so he said little about them. Even then, however, he did strongly advocate eating only natural, unprocessed foods. One example: he recommended eating only unsulfured dried fruits.
- Alcohol, nicotine, and recreational drugs will work against your desire to experience Spirit, as well as against your personal freedom. If you consume such substances, use your spiritual aspirations as incentives to cut down on—or better still, end—those habits.

- Eat only at regular times—and not too late at night. If you're not hungry at one of those times, don't eat. If you're hungry, eat moderately. If you're just a little bit hungry, eat just a little bit.
- Don't be hypnotized by the thought of three meals a day; skip a meal now and then to give your body a rest from digesting food. If you don't do much manual labor, then two meals might be plenty on most days. Regular fasting, too, is highly beneficial for most people.
- Pray before eating. Bless your food, and give thanks for it. The point is not only to show appropriate gratitude: yogis say that gratitude and appreciation will enhance your body's ability to assimilate the nutrients in your food.

Apply It to Your Life

Choose one aspect of your diet that needs improvement. Maybe you know that you should eat more fresh fruits and vegetables, or less animal flesh, or less junk food, or … ahem … drink fewer sodas or coffees. Give it a try. Conduct the experiment: create a specific plan, and stick with it despite any initial resistance from your body or mind. If, after a couple weeks, you feel at least as good as you did before—and you'll likely feel much better than you did before—make that change a part of your normal diet. Then try improving another aspect of your diet. It's a simple and effective approach: experiment, learn, revise, repeat.

Of course, you'll want to conduct your experiment intelligently, in a balanced and healthy way. To learn how to do that, and to explore healthier dietary patterns in general, see "Yogic Health, Diet & Cooking" in Appendix B: Further Exploration.

7.6—LIGHTEN UP

Is all this too much? Please remember: it's just a menu of options. Try out any that seem to have potential for you, one or two at a time, at a pace that works for you, and closely monitor your joy level. Let joy always be your barometer of what works: if the joy level plummets, you've gone too far—for now, anyway. Grim determination and self-deprivation rarely lead to enjoyment—and without enjoyment, you'll become resentful or abandon the experiment.

Becoming overly serious is just another example of being out of balance, but this imbalance deserves separate mention. To put it simply, you're much more likely to experience divine joy if you're joyful!

Apply It to Your Life

There are many ways to cultivate joy. As I mentioned above, it helps to spend time with joyful people, or in places that inspire you to feel joy. When doing things you enjoy, *consciously* enjoy doing them—it's practice for doing joyfully other things that you might not otherwise enjoy. Practice joyfulness in mundane everyday activities: while you brush your teeth, wash dishes, drive your car, or exercise. Practice being joyful as a service to others; everyone likes to be around an upbeat person. All of this strengthens your ability to be joyful in any circumstance.

Here's another way to cultivate joy: read one funny story every day. In fact, Paramhansa Yogananda specifically recommended doing so. You might not expect a great spiritual teacher to champion such a seemingly trivial thing, but humor (at least when it's kindly, not sarcastic or judgmental) truly is an aid to spiritual growth, for it relaxes you and gives you a healthier perspective on other people, on events, *and on yourself.* All this naturally helps you move toward balance, harmony, and joy.

For example, at Ananda Village (the ashram where I live) we have a long-standing tradition of enjoying the short stories of P.G. Wodehouse, the famous English humorist. Sometimes a group of residents will stage an informal "readers' theater" production. Sometimes we listen to Swami Kriyananda read a story aloud. And sometimes it's fun simply to curl up on the couch and read Wodehouse. You won't get far in a Wodehouse story without a good chuckle; more than likely, you'll have to stop and laugh out loud. Wodehouse never uses put-down humor. His stories are delightful perspectives on the human comedy, amusing all and offending no one.

Other good sources of uplifting humor include:

- Funny, violence-free movies—from classics with the Marx Brothers or Laurel & Hardy, to some good recent ones
- Cleverly funny animated TV shows or movies—oldies such as *The Rocky & Bullwinkle Show*, *The Bugs Bunny Show*, *The Road Runner Show*, and *The Tom & Jerry Show*; also certain recent full-length animated movies by Pixar or DreamWorks
- Books of clean, non-sarcastic jokes
- Books that are compilations of certain classic comic strips, such as *Peanuts*, *Calvin & Hobbes*, *The Far Side*

And on a regular basis simply have a good laugh, just for the sheer joy of laughing.

Chapter
EIGHT

Two More Aids
on the Journey

*Keep your spine ever straight: It is the channel through which
energy flows up to the brain. If that upward flow is weakened
or impeded, your power to meet life's challenges will diminish.
Truthfulness demands an attitude of firmness, integrity, and clear
vision. These virtues all depend on the upward flow of energy in
the spine.*

—SWAMI KRIYANANDA

I'll conclude by briefly mentioning two more key aspects of Yoga. Both are closely interwoven with the practice of techniques as well as with the yogic lifestyle. The first one—right attitude—has been part of this book from the beginning, but there are a few more points to make.

8.1—RIGHT ATTITUDE

Your awareness rises—or not—through not only *what* you do, but also *how* you do it: attitude is the most powerful of all spiritual tools. It is the key factor in success or failure in every endeavor, whether inner or outer. Techniques will aid spiritual growth only to the extent that you practice them with right attitude.

Right attitude isn't about moral judgments or merely being a nice person: what makes an attitude right is that it aligns you with your own true nature. Only then can you transcend ego-consciousness and move toward soul-consciousness. Both the Bhagavad Gita and the Yoga Sutras strongly emphasize many such attitudes: humility, kindness, compassion, honesty, generosity, self-control, nonattachment, devotion, contentment, fearlessness, and a host of others.

Stop for a moment and re-read that list of attitudes. Try to *feel* how each one takes you away from the egoic tendency to identify with your body, your personality, your likes and dislikes, and helps you align with the Divine. Some expand your circle of caring, so it's not "all about me." Some affirm that your happiness doesn't depend on ego-gratification or any external circumstance. Others help you avoid protecting or reinforcing the ego. Still others affirm a commitment to a reality greater than the ego. Each one brings a sense of relaxation, expansion, and freedom.

Take this into your daily life: in any given situation, try to adopt an attitude that will give you that expansive sense of freedom. It's usually easy to think of one, though not always easy to adopt it. It's easier, however, if you've previously strengthened the attitude within you. Here are a few ways to do that:

- In earlier chapters I've emphasized how each yogic technique promotes a positive attitude of mind. Ananda Yoga®, with its added power of asana affirmations and working directly with energy, amplifies that effect. Every time you practice, you're strengthening right attitudes—and the deeper you practice, the stronger those attitudes will be.

- Spend time with people who have right attitudes. Don't merely try to take from them; that will tend to deplete them, and it doesn't help you much. You'll draw much more if you *attune* yourself to them, and if there's an exchange of energy: serve them somehow, do a small favor, or silently appreciate and bless them. Then their magnetism will naturally strengthen your own.

- In daily life, whenever you succeed in having a right attitude in a challenging situation, celebrate your victory over the temptation to be small, limited, and separate. Savor the feeling of freedom that it brings. This reinforces that right attitude, making it more likely that you'll succeed next time too.

- What if you don't succeed in having a right attitude? Don't use the energy of regret to beat yourself up. Rather, channel any such energy in a positive direction: affirm with deep determination, "I *will* succeed next time!" That, too, will strengthen the attitude.

Whether on the mat or in everyday life, strengthening right attitude is an adventure in reclaiming your soul freedom. It's not an esoteric process; the opportunities are right in front of you, moment to moment. All you need to do is take advantage of the opportunities as they arise.

8.2—A GUIDE FOR THE JOURNEY

A great deal of spiritual growth can take place through our own efforts, and through keeping the company of others who share our aspirations. However, great masters of Yoga maintain that if we aspire to the pinnacle of human potential—Self-realization—we need a guru. A *guru* (literally, dispeller of darkness) is not just another teacher. A guru is one who has transcended ego-identification, and attained not only Self-realization, but also the divine power to help others do the same.

The idea of a guru is a sticking point for many people. Some think that they don't need a guru in order to achieve union with the Infinite. Others fear that a guru will exploit them, take away their free will, make them dependent, or mislead them in some way.

Suppose, however, that you want to be a mountain climber. You could easily find a website that outlines the basic principles, buy some equipment recommended there, and try it on your own. You might well succeed in some easy climbs.

But if you want to climb challenging mountains, wouldn't it be wiser to learn directly from an expert climber? He or she can help you develop your abilities, minimize the risks, and overcome your fears and limitations. Working with an expert will give you the freedom to do more, not less.

It's wiser still to seek expert help with climbing the mountain of your spiritual aspirations. That journey is far more ambitious and promises far more fulfillment—and yes, can be more perilous—than climbing outward mountains. The guru's job is to provide that help. The guru won't do the work for you, but he or she will help you build the strength and give you the support to make the climb. As Paramhansa Yogananda put it:

> The purpose of the guru is not to weaken your will. It is to teach you secrets of developing your inner power, until you can stand unshaken amidst the crash of breaking worlds.

I'm not urging you to rush out and find a guru if you don't already have one. No one should try to convince you to do that; the urge must come from within you. As time passes and you climb farther up your mountain, you'll realize that it's higher than you'd imagined—which is to say, your own potential is greater than you'd imagined. The day will come when you realize that your aspirations are both urgent and far beyond your capacity to attain them. You'll know then that you need help.

Perhaps that time is now, or perhaps it's yet to come. In any case, great yogis say that God *wants* to help us, and *will* help us once our own efforts have prepared us to receive and cooperate with that help. As the Indian scriptures say, "When the disciple is ready, the guru appears."

Then Yoga *really* begins to happen.

Appendix A

Origins of Ananda Yoga

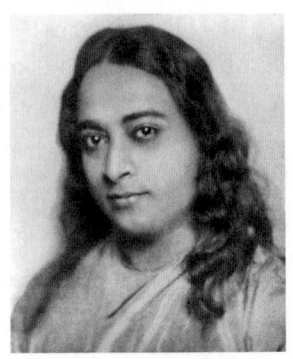

Paramhansa Yogananda

Ananda Yoga® comes from the teachings of PARAMHANSA YOGANANDA, author of the highly acclaimed book, *Autobiography of a Yogi*. He was the first great master of Yoga to make his home in the West, where he lived from 1920 until his passing in 1952. His mission in coming to the West was twofold: to share the scientific techniques of Yoga, in which India has specialized over the millennia; and to show that the original teachings of Yoga (as given by Krishna in the Bhagavad Gita) and the original teachings of Christianity (as given by Jesus) are, behind all the outward trappings, essentially the same. By extension, one can easily see that the differences among all true spiritual teachings are differences of emphasis and of outward practices; the inward essence is the same.

Although Yogananda taught Hatha Yoga techniques to some of his close disciples, he didn't teach Hatha publicly, nor did he strongly emphasize it; he called it "useful, but not essential." His primary focus was meditation, the central technique of all Yoga. It was his disciple, SWAMI KRIYANANDA, who organized Yogananda's approach to Hatha Yoga into a specific system.

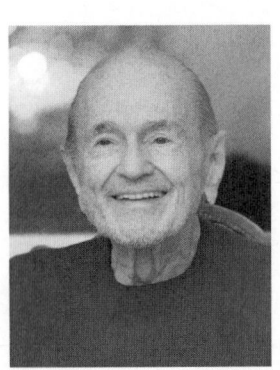

Swami Kriyananda

Kriyananda, an American born in Romania and raised in Europe, became Yogananda's disciple in 1948, and lived with the master until Yogananda's passing. Under Yogananda's direct supervision, he would often demonstrate for guests and visitors the master's approach to asanas.

Kriyananda observed that, even among his fellow disciples, the prevailing perspective on the asanas was physical: toning of muscles, stimulation of glands, etc. Yogananda had little interest in the physical aspect, though he acknowledged that it was beneficial. Kriyananda recalls his own thoughts at that time:

This physical emphasis isn't Master's [Yogananda's] teachings! Hatha Yoga *must* have another benefit. It can't be just pressing on your thyroid gland to flush it out, and things like that. That would no doubt be a part of it, but that's not what Master came to teach. And it can't be Yoga if that's all it is. It may be a good physical exercise, but Yoga has a purpose, and the fact that Hatha Yoga is the physical branch of Raja Yoga means that the purpose of Hatha Yoga has to be spiritual; it can't be just to give you a good body.

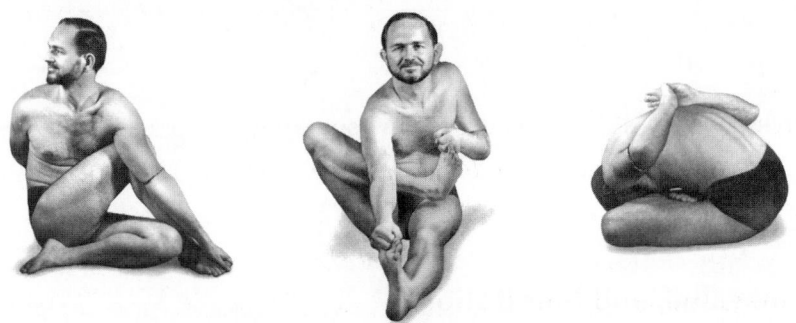

Swami Kriyananda practicing Ananda Yoga

After Yogananda's *mahasamadhi* (his conscious exit from the body), Kriyananda developed this aspect of his guru's teaching into the comprehensive system known as Ananda Yoga for Higher Awareness (or more concisely, Ananda Yoga), described in his seminal book, *Ananda Yoga for Higher Awareness*. Although it was he who formalized the Ananda approach, Kriyananda emphasized that "Ananda Yoga is Master's system, not mine."

Kriyananda later founded the worldwide Ananda movement (Ananda.org), dedicated to living and spreading the nonsectarian spiritual teachings of Paramhansa Yogananda. Its main location is Ananda Village, a thriving Northern California community of more than 200 dedicated yogis. Founded in 1968, Ananda Village is a living laboratory for—and shining example of—the practicality and effectiveness of Yoga for living a happy, successful, God-centered life. There are additional Ananda communities and teaching centers in the United States (California, Washington, and Oregon), Italy, and India. The principles of Yoga guide the lives of the many hundreds of residents of these communities. Visit Ananda.org for more information.

If you want to *experience* Yoga as a complete way of life, and learn how to bring it into your own life, wherever you may live, you can get it all at Ananda's year-round spiritual retreat facility, The Expanding Light (ExpandingLight.org) at Ananda Village.

Appendix B

Further Exploration

The resources below will take you deeper in your study and practice of spiritual Hatha Yoga as well as the greater science of Yoga. All are available at CrystalClarity.com except where noted.

Asana, Pranayama, and Meditation

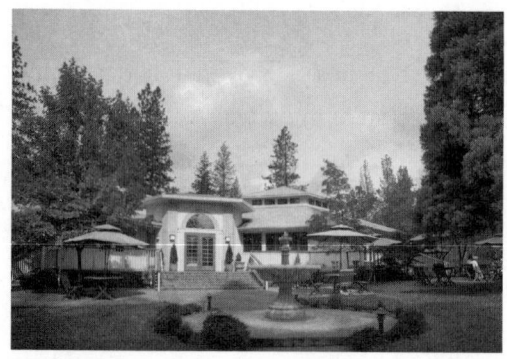
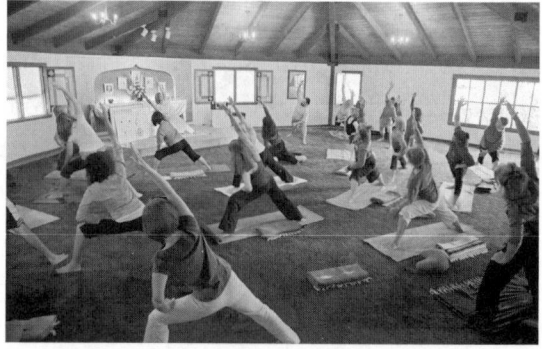

Ananda's Northern California spiritual retreat facility, The Expanding Light (Expanding-Light.org), offers, among its many programs, systematic training in Ananda Yoga®, meditation, and yoga therapy. Private lessons are also available.

Nayaswami Gyandev and other Ananda teachers have produced a variety of Ananda Yoga DVD's, including *The Ananda Yoga Series*, in which Gyandev leads 48 Ananda Yoga classes that explore many aspects of the spiritual life—experientially, through asana, pranayama, and meditation. For details, visit AnandaYoga.org, where you'll also find an audio Sanskrit pronunciation guide and instructional video clips for the asanas.

For information on Kriya Yoga, the highest meditation technique brought to the West by Paramhansa Yogananda, visit Ananda.org/kriya-yoga.

Also recommended:

- *Yoga to Awaken the Chakras*, a DVD by Gyandev McCord

- *Yoga for Busy People*, a DVD by Gyandev McCord

- *Lessons in Meditation*, a book/CD/DVD collection

- *How to Meditate*, a book by Jyotish Novak

- *Meditation for Inner Peace*, a CD by Diksha McCord (WaysToFreedom.com)

- *Pranayama for Deeper Meditation*, a two-CD set by Nayaswami Gyandev (WaysToFreedom.com)

- Distance learning through OnlineWithAnanda.org

Energization Exercises

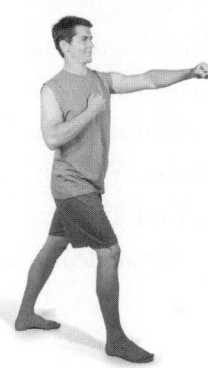

Paramhansa Yogananda designed this innovative system to recharge the body with life-force and to teach greater awareness of and control over that energy, ultimately bringing the practitioner to a perception of the body *as* energy. As a new expression of ancient Yoga principles, this system is one of Yogananda's primary contributions to the field of Yoga. Energization is best learned in person at The Expanding Light Retreat (ExpandingLight.org) or at one of Ananda's other teaching centers (visit AnandaYoga.org for locations). You can also learn via the *Energization* DVD, *Energization* booklet, or Volume 2 of *The Ananda Yoga Series* on DVD (AnandaYoga.org).

Props for Hatha Yoga and Meditation

Asana blankets, straps, cushions, and meditation benches are available at AnandaYoga.org.

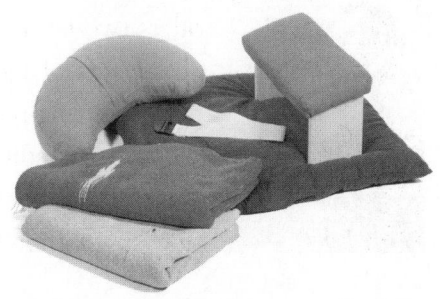

Teacher Training and Continuing Education

The Expanding Light Retreat offers professional teacher training in three areas: Ananda Yoga, Ananda Yoga Therapy, and Meditation. All three programs include comprehensive training, mentored practice teaching, and full immersion in the Yoga lifestyle:

Ananda Yoga Teacher Training (Levels 1 & 2)

If you'd like to teach spiritual Hatha Yoga—or simply deepen your experience of it—consider Ananda's 200- and 500-hour Yoga Teacher Trainings. Level 1 (200 hours) focuses primarily on asana and meditation. Level 2 (300 hours after Level 1) emphasizes advanced asana and pranayama, teaching meditation, deeper topics in Yoga philosophy, adapting asanas for individual needs, spiritual counselor training, and personal spiritual growth. Teachers of other styles can enter the advanced (Level 2) teacher training, without doing Ananda's full 200-hour training, via the Bridge to Ananda Yoga program. Ananda's Level 1 & 2 YTTs are registered with Yoga Alliance at 200 and 500 hours, respectively. (ExpandingLight.org/aytt)

Ananda Yoga Therapy Training (Levels 1 & 2)

Learn to apply the principles and techniques of Yoga to help people with injuries or illness by addressing each person at *all* levels of being: physical, mental, emotional, and spiritual. Level 1 includes client assessment, musculoskeletal therapy, Ayurveda, pranayama, adapting asanas for individual needs, healing at a distance, teaching meditation and restorative yoga, and a variety of specialty training areas. The prerequisite is Yoga Alliance RYT 200. Level 1 Yoga Therapy graduates can register as RYT 500. Ananda's Level 2 Yoga Therapy Training adds meditation therapy training, spiritual counselor training, radiant health teacher training, and additional specialty areas. (ExpandingLight.org/ytx)

Ananda Meditation Teacher Training (Levels 1 & 2)

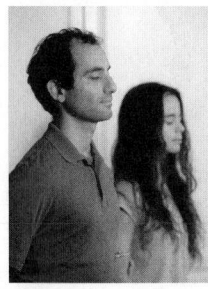

To help you serve the growing demand for learning to meditate, Ananda offers two levels of meditation teacher certification: Level 1 focuses on all aspects of meditation—from helping each student find his or her perfect sitting position, to learning to teach a variety of tools and techniques for meditation. Level 2 explores meditation in more depth (in your personal practice as well as in teaching deeper aspects of meditation) in addition to training you to serve others through spiritual counseling, stress management training, working with the chakras, and meditation therapy. (ExpandingLight.org/mtt)

Yoga Teacher Support Center

This is an online source of articles and inspiration that will support and instruct both teachers and students of Hatha Yoga. (ExpandingLight.org/ytsc)

Raja Yoga, Chakras, and Yoga Philosophy

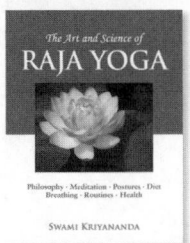 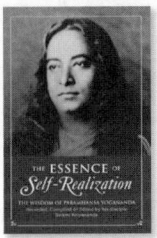 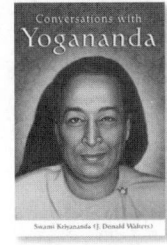 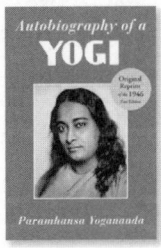 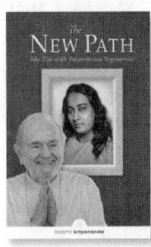

To explore more deeply the broader teachings of Yoga, read Swami Kriyananda's comprehensive book, *The Art and Science of Raja Yoga*. Another excellent source is Kriyananda's *Demystifying Patanjali: The Yoga Sutras (Aphorisms)*.

For more information on the chakras, read *Chakras for Starters: Unlock the Hidden Doors to Peace & Well-Being* by Savitri Simpson.

You'll find additional insights into Yoga in the original edition of Yogananda's classic, *Autobiography of a Yogi*; in Swami Kriyananda's compilations of quotations by Yogananda (*The Essence of Self-Realization* and *Conversations with Yogananda*); and in Kriyananda's own autobiography, *The New Path*.

Right Attitude and Affirmation

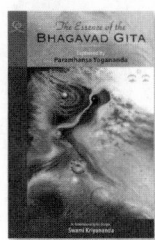 For a deeper, practical exploration of the psychological and spiritual dimensions of right attitude, read *The Essence of the Bhagavad Gita* and *The Art and Science of Raja Yoga*, both by Swami Kriyananda.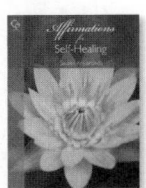

For more on the yogic science of affirmation, read *Affirmations for Self-Healing* and *The Art and Science of Raja Yoga*, both by Swami Kriyananda (CrystalClarity.com), as well as *Scientific Healing Affirmations* by Paramhansa Yogananda (Self-Realization Fellowship).

Yogic Health, Diet & Cooking

You'll find a compilation of Paramhansa Yogananda's writings on health and diet in the book, *How to Achieve Glowing Health and Vitality*. For personal training in applying these principles to your life, take the Ananda Holistic Health Training course at The Expanding Light Retreat (ExpandingLight. org).

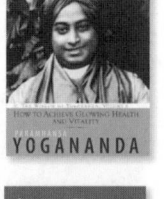

Vegetarian Cooking for Starters, by Blanche (Diksha) Agassy McCord, is an excellent primer on vegetarian diet, with many simple recipes. She has also written a popular vegetarian/vegan cookbook: *Global Kitchen*.

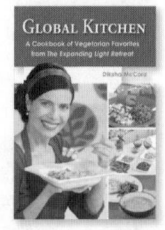

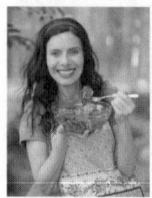

Diksha has created an online, hands-on video series, "Vegetarian Cooking for Health & Vitality." Topics range from seasonal meals to holiday meals to specialty areas such as breads, teas, herbs & spices, desserts, and more. For details, visit the online learning section of ExpandingLight.org.

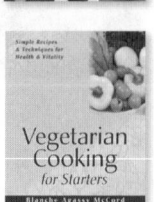

Cultivating Your Divine Connection

Here are several excellent books that explore the keys to developing an intimate, personal relationship with Spirit:

- *How You Can Talk with God*, Paramhansa Yogananda (Self-Realization Fellowship)
- *Practicing His Presence*, letters by Brother Lawrence and Frank Laubach (SeedSowers)
- *The Way of a Pilgrim*, translated by R.M. French (Harper Collins)

Glossary

Agya chakra[15] (*agya* **means "perceive"; also "command"**)—the sixth chakra. Its positive pole is the spiritual eye, and its negative pole is the astral medulla oblongata.

Anahata chakra (*anahata* **means "unstruck"**)—the fourth chakra, located in the center of the chest opposite the physical heart. It's the seat of love, compassion, generosity, kindness, and intuitive feeling, the faculty with which one perceives reality as it truly is—and oneself as one truly is: the soul, not the ego.

Asana—position of the body. Usually it refers to one of the Hatha Yoga postures.

Astral body—the subtle body composed of energy. It creates, sustains, and roughly resembles the physical body.

Astral breath—the upward and downward flows of energy in the astral spine as you inhale and exhale, respectively.

Astral spine—the main pathway through which prana (subtle energy) flows to the brain. The astral spine runs through the center of the body, just in front of the physical spinal column: from the tip of the tailbone to the medulla oblongata at the base of the brain, then forward and up to the spiritual eye.

Bandha—a yoga technique in which you close or tighten a certain area of the body, thereby concentrating energy in a particular location and/or causing energy to move in a particular direction.

Chakra—any of the astral body's seven main energy centers. Located in the astral spine, the chakras govern all bodily functions. Their energies also both influence and reflect your state of mind, which makes them central to the process of raising your awareness.

---

[15] One sees several different transliterations of a certain Sanskrit consonant that has no English equivalent: *gy* (as in *agya*), *jn* (*ajna*), and *jñ* (*ajña*). I use the *gy* transliteration, which, according to Paramhansa Yogananda, leads the English speaker to a pronunciation—a hard "g" as in "good"—that, while not perfect, is closer to the ancient Sanskrit.

Ego—the soul, the Infinite Self, identified with the body and personality.

Guru—"dispeller of darkness," one who has transcended ego-identification and attained not only Self-realization, but also the divine power to help others do the same.

Hatha Yoga—the physical branch of Yoga. Literally, it translates as union of the *ha* (solar) and *tha* (lunar) energies in the spine, the rising and descending currents that cause physical inhalations and exhalations. Hatha Yoga includes asanas, pranayamas, bandhas, and mudras; the Ananda Yoga® expression of Hatha Yoga also emphasizes Paramhansa Yogananda's Energization Exercises and, above all, meditation.

Medulla oblongata—The physical medulla oblongata is located where the spinal cord meets the brain. Its astral counterpart is the negative pole of the agya chakra. The astral medulla oblongata is the primary point through which prana enters the body. It's also the seat of ego-consciousness: the notion that you're separate from all other beings, and from Spirit.

Mudra—a special position or action of certain body part(s), designed to awaken spiritual energies and/or to redirect energy.

Prana—the subtle energy (life-force) that animates the physical body.

Pranayama—energy-control. Although it most commonly refers to breath-control techniques, pranayama is a broad category of techniques that control energy in various ways: e.g., bandhas, mudras, and Paramhansa Yogananda's Energization Exercises, as well as breath-control techniques.

Raja Yoga—"royal yoga," the overall spiritual science of Yoga, of which Hatha Yoga is the physical branch (and only a small part of the whole). Raja Yoga includes a spectrum of traditional approaches (wisdom, devotion, service, technique) to Self-realization, with meditation as the supreme guide.

Self-realization—the true goal of Yoga: the direct and enduring experience of your eternal oneness with all creation and with Spirit beyond creation. You may or may not aspire to Self-realization, but you certainly aspire to lasting happiness, and the route that leads to lasting happiness leads ultimately to Self-realization.

Sitbones (aka sitting bones, sitzbones)—the two bony prominences where the hamstring muscles attach to the pelvis. These are the two places that get sore when you sit too long on a hard surface.

Spiritual eye (aka third eye)—the positive pole of the agya chakra. Located just interior to the point between the eyebrows, in the forehead, it is the seat of willpower, concentration, reason, joy, and superconsciousness. The highest purpose of Hatha Yoga is to bring energy to the spiritual eye to help the yogi toward the experience of superconsciousness.

Straight spine (aka neutral spine)—the physical spinal column in its healthy, natural curves: an inward curve near waist level, an outward curve in the chest region, and an inward curve through the neck. The straighter your physical spine, the more open your astral spine will be, and thus the easier it will be for energy to flow to the brain.

Subtle gravity—a force that acts upon energy in the same way that physical gravity acts upon the body: when you're upright, subtle gravity pulls your energy downward, toward the base of your spine, and so inclines you toward materialistic consciousness. Subtle gravity is therefore a spiritual adversary when your body is in an upright position; but when your spine is upside down (as in an inverted asana), that same force becomes a spiritual ally: it draws energy toward your brain and thereby helps to raise your consciousness.

Superconsciousness (aka soul-consciousness)—a heightened state of awareness in which you perceive the unity of all things and all beings.

Tuck the pelvis (aka posteriorly tilt the pelvis, retrovert the pelvis)— Tilt the pelvis so that its top rim moves backward, thereby flattening the natural inward curve of your lumbar (lower) spine. This movement helps you avoid over-curving the lumbar spine (i.e., bending it backward too sharply) in certain asanas. In some asanas, instead of thinking in terms of moving the pelvis, it may feel more natural to accomplish this by drawing the navel toward the spine, or by lengthening the tailbone away from the lower back, or by drawing the pubis toward the navel.

Index of Techniques

This index includes all the techniques described in this book: asanas (with their Ananda Yoga® affirmations), pranayamas, bandhas, mudras, and meditation. It's divided into two listings: the first is alphabetical by Sanskrit name, and the second is alphabetical by English name. Asana affirmations appear in italics below each asana's name.

ALPHABETICAL BY SANSKRIT NAME

ALPHABETICAL BY ENGLISH NAME

(Seated) Mountain Pose—Parvatasana, 123

"My thoughts and energy rise up to touch the sky."

(Standing) Mountain Pose—Tadasana, 58

"I stand ready to obey Thy least command."

Peacock Feather Pose—
Pincha Mayurasana, 134

"The Infinite Light cascades through my spine."

Peacock Pose—Mayurasana, 119

[Use the awakened energy itself as your affirmation.]

Perfect Pose—Siddhasana, 144

"I set ablaze the fire of inner joy."

Plow Pose—Halasana, 129

"New life, new consciousness now flood my brain!"

Posterior-Stretching Pose—
Paschimotanasana, 85

"I am safe. I am sound. All good things come to me; they give me peace!"

Pulling-the-Bow Pose—
Akarshana Dhanurasana, 113

"With shafts of will I pierce the heart of worries."

Root Lock—Mula Bandha, 165

Royal Pigeon Pose—Rajakapotasana, 102

"I rise above all thought of past and future, into the Eternal Now."

Seated Angle Pose—
Upavistha Konasana, 88

"I welcome every opportunity for further growth."

Shoulderstand—Sarvangasana, 126

"God's peace now floods my being."

Side Angle Pose—Parsvakonasana, 78

"I am a fountain of boundless energy and power!"

**Side Stretching Pose
(aka Pyramid Pose)**—Parsvotanasana, 69

"I offer myself fully into the flow of grace."

Simple Inverted Pose—Viparita Karani, 128

"Awake, my sleeping powers, awake!"

Stomach Lift—Uddiyana Bandha, 166

Sun Salutation—Surya Namaskar, 80

"Salutations to the sun, to the awakening light within, to the dawning of higher consciousness in all beings."

Supine Firm Pose—Supta Vajrasana, 92

"Energetic movement or unmoving peace: The choice is mine alone! The choice is mine!"

About the Author

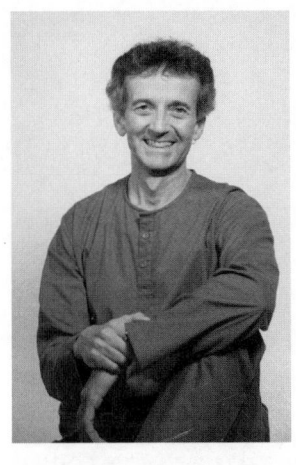

NAYASWAMI[16] GYANDEV (RICHARD) MCCORD, PHD, E-RYT 500 is the director of Ananda Yoga® and Ananda Yoga Teacher Training. He has taught Ananda Yoga, as well as all aspects of its parent science, Raja Yoga, since 1983. He is a co-founder and long-time board member of Yoga Alliance, the nonprofit organization that sets minimum standards for the training of teachers in the U.S.

Gyandev has produced two Ananda Yoga DVD's—*Yoga for Busy People* and *Yoga to Awaken the Chakras*—as well as the 12 volumes (48 classes) of *The Ananda Yoga Series*, also on DVD. He has co-authored two books with Dr. Peter Van Houten—*Yoga Therapy for Overcoming Insomnia* and *Yoga Therapy for Relieving Headaches*. All are available at CrystalClarity.org.

He has also authored two booklets—*Guide to the Mahabharata and Life of Sri Krishna* and *A Concise Bhagavad Gita*—as well as a number of audio CD's, including *Pranayama for Deeper Meditation*, *Ease into Sleep*, *Connect with Spirit*, *Magnetize Your Life*, and *Dance of Divinity*. All these are available at his personal website, WaysToFreedom.com.

Gyandev has lived at Ananda Village in Northern California since 1984. He and his wife, Nayaswami Diksha, serve as ministers and teachers at The Expanding Light (ExpandingLight.org), Ananda's retreat center. They also lead workshops in many locations around the world.

Gyandev received his B.A. in Mathematics from Carleton College, and his M.S. and Ph.D. in Operations Research (an area of applied mathematics) from Stanford University.

---

[16] For information on the Nayaswami Order, a new movement in renunciation, visit nayaswami.org, or see the book, *A Renunciate Order for the New Age* (CrystalClarity.com).

CRYSTAL CLARITY PUBLISHERS

Crystal Clarity Publishers offers additional resources to assist you in your spiritual journey, including many other books, a wide variety of inspirational and relaxation music composed by Swami Kriyananda, and yoga and meditation videos. To see a complete listing of our products, contact us for a print catalog or see our website: www.crystalclarity.com

Crystal Clarity Publishers
14618 Tyler Foote Rd., Nevada City, CA 95959
TOLL FREE: 800.424.1055 or 530.478.7600 / FAX: 530.478.7610
EMAIL: clarity@crystalclarity.com

ANANDA WORLDWIDE

Ananda Sangha, a worldwide organization founded by Swami Kriyananda, offers spiritual support and resources based on the teachings of Paramhansa Yogananda. There are Ananda spiritual communities in Nevada City, Sacramento, Palo Alto, and Los Angeles, California; Seattle, Washington; Portland and Laurelwood, Oregon; as well as a retreat center and European community in Assisi, Italy, and communities near New Delhi and Pune, India. Ananda supports more than 140 meditation groups worldwide.

For more information about Ananda Sangha communities or meditation
groups near you, please call 530.478.7560 or visit www.ananda.org

THE EXPANDING LIGHT

Ananda's guest retreat, The Expanding Light, offers a varied, year-round schedule of classes and workshops on yoga, meditation, and spiritual practice. You may also come for a relaxed personal renewal, participating in ongoing activities as much or as little as you wish. The beautiful serene mountain setting, supportive staff, and delicious vegetarian food provide an ideal environment for a truly meaningful, spiritual vacation.

For more information, please call 800.346.5350
or visit www.expandinglight.org